THE PASTOR AND THE PATIENT

In memory of
Dr. William F. Jacobs,
Physician, Teacher
and Constant Searcher

The Pastor
and the Patient

*an informal guide to
new directions in medical ethics*

by
William Jacobs

PAULIST PRESS
New York / Paramus / Toronto

Library of Congress
Catalog Card Number: 73-85727

ISBN 0-8091-1789-4

Published by Paulist Press
Editorial Office: 1865 Broadway, N.Y., N.Y. 10023
Business Office: 400 Sette Drive, Paramus, N.J. 07652

Printed and bound in the
United States of America

Contents

SPECIAL ACKNOWLEDGMENTS

Particular thanks are due to Rev. Anthony Kosnik, SS. Cyril and Methodius Seminary; Drs. Andre Hellegers and Warren Reich of the John F. Kennedy Center for Bioethics; Dr. Charles McCarthy, National Institutes of Health, and to Sr. Mary Janice Belen, R.S.M., St. Lawrence Hospital, Lansing, Michigan and to many others in the health care and general academic fields for inspiration, aid and counsel in the preparation of this book. It should be freely acknowledged that the work of Dr. Paul Ramsey, particularly as published in *The Patient as Person* and *Fabricated Man* (Yale University Press), provided a base for much of the thinking reflected in the pages to follow. Special gratitude is due my wife, Gloria Jacobs, R.N.

Introduction

It used to be, or at least we thought at the time that it was, a time of security and relative certainty, with the possibility of fairly straight, uncomplicated answers to most problems.

These answers came from various sources; perhaps the Church was the first. Then, as time went on, the "godlike" stature of the physician increased and answers which were rarely challenged came from him. More and more we looked to a philosophy of science and then a religion of science, wherein we believed that if we didn't have a ready answer just then, it was just around the corner. In recent years a new group of answer-providers—the administrative class—has become prominent in every phase of our lives.

Unfortunately, the complexities of society, the explosion of knowledge, the rejection of old concepts held largely for their own sake, and any number of other factors have taken away that kind of reasonably sure, reasonably sound, comforting answer that could be offered to a man, a woman or couple facing a difficult decision. Nowhere is this more evident than in the field of medical ethics and morality.

In fact, merely approaching medical ethics and morality from a theoretical point of view has accomplished relatively little except in highly specialized circles. Medical personnel for the most part are concerned with what *can* be done rather than with what *should* be done. The administrators have all but administered us right out of business and the answers which they give rarely smack of certainty in any direction.

Scientific research, the place where we all look for ultimate answers and solutions, has in fact provided us with more problems. The ordinary medical decision made today is perhaps a hundred times more complex than it would have been even twenty years ago.

Now translate this into the situation of the ordinary working priest, whether hospital chaplain, parish priest, or any other priest called upon to counsel patients or professional personnel on the morality of some practice or procedure which is being considered. He starts out with great handicaps, having been led to believe earlier in his life that there were some fairly simple and direct solutions. Even if he has kept up-to-date on moral theology and realizes that there are a lot fewer absolutes than he once believed, he isn't left in a very strong position. He rarely feels confidence in the advice that he gives and this is a good thing because this kind of advice can rarely be given with strong confidence by any one person. Decisions in the medical moral field involve the thinking, experience and hard and fast know-how of any number of persons in any number of specialities. The man engaged in pastoral work is reduced or promoted, depending on how you look at it, to being a sort of mediator, the man who keeps himself as informed as possible and aids people in reaching the best possible judgments in terms of their human needs and the demands of a legitimate incarnational and total morality.

It is to these men that this book is directed, although it may have value to others. They cannot be constantly informed of every development in medicine or in the various phases of medical and biological research which will affect present and future moral questions. They cannot rely on the authority of their "grace of state" to mandate a decision to persons who may very well have already made the decision and are only in the pastoral offices for the purpose of confirmation of their own judgment.

Beyond that, no matter how good a theologian or how good a medical moral theologian he may be, the man in the pastoral situation realizes quite quickly that there are areas where morality and ethics cross pastoral ministry in such a way as to cause conflicts which create what appear to be dilemmas. Working out solutions is no small task.

This book, of course, cannot attempt to provide all of the answers in advance. It can be as up-to-date as possible on what's going on in the field and it can help to provide guidance as to attitudes which the man in a pastoral situation can have in aiding his clients or parishioners to make truly moral decisions. We are not dealing purely with ethics or morality but also with pastoral ministry and we have to realize a very important thing. There was a time when we assumed that the final word on the legitimacy of a medical action would come from the Church. But today a much more common view is that the Church is one of several bodies or agencies with a right and obligation to address itself to a given ethical or moral question. Short of moral situations on which there is truly unbending Church teaching, the Church must be viewed, at least in the decision-making process, as one voice, representing God, but not always positive of the will of God, one voice trying to find a Christian solution to a human problem and to guide afflicted persons toward whatever treatment they may need within a Christian moral context.

However, in the practical order the prudential judgments of competent physicians must also be considered; so must the views of various legislative bodies; so must the ideas of various neighborhood or regional groups. The Church can no longer stand alone as the sole source of the sole answer to the problem. This certainly does not make it easier for the man in the pastoral role. It places upon him the same kind of added painful responsibility that our newer approaches to morality in general have placed on the ordinary person living an ordinary life. Certainly he will have moments of doubt, even moments of anguish. It would seem that the most that could be expected of him would be his best possible efforts to keep informed, to think clearly, to guide the thinking process of those who consult him without imposing his judgments upon them, and, in all cases, to give them support and encouragement in whatever course they follow, even when he considers that course to be sinful. After all his primary call is to minister to sinners not just to approve the righteous.

We won't be terribly concerned here with the kind of cheap legalism that concerns itself with the use of a cannula to remove the menstrual material of a woman who is a few days past her period without first attempting to determine whether or not conception has occurred. Such a procedure is inexpensive and relatively convenient and will circumvent most anti-abortion laws that still exist after Supreme Court decisions and the

inevitable legal hassles that follow. The pastoral counselor is bound to consider the preservation of human
life that is at least potentially present from the moment
of conception. But the simple removing of material
without determining whether the period delay had
anything to do with pregnancy is not a question with
which he need concern himself very much.

What he needs is constantly increasing knowledge,
constantly increasing humanity and a recognition of
the constantly increasing need of ordinary people for
support and encouragement as they live through a
very difficult time. Very few of these people, even those
who would be labeled conservative, are adhering to
static positions these days. When they make a judgment on a moral matter they make it, as they should,
after considerable reflection. What they want from the
Church is not so much a legalistic stamp of approval
but a Christlike assistance in forming the most moral
judgment of which they are capable and the living out
of that.

Regrettably, many things will happen between now
and the ultimate publication of this book which will
raise even more questions and which may change certain
attitudes and directions of judgment expressed in these
pages. This is the very nature of the situation. During
the long months spent writing the book, I have run
into countless situations where I asked medical questions for which I could receive no adequate medical
answer. Similarly, in consultation with some of the
finest moralists in the country, I have raised many
questions which received, at most, tentative or speculative answers. It is this kind of situation with which
the man in pastoral life must deal. About all he can
do about it is think a lot, pray a lot, and try very hard.

1. What's New?

The answer to the question raised in the title of this chapter is: Practically everything.

It is a widely used truism that science and technology have proceeded at a gallop in our time, while ethics and morality have barely crawled forward. Nowhere is the gap more evident than in the field of medical ethics and the ethics of related fields. The guidelines issued by the American Bishops in November of 1971, which make up Appendix I of this book, were referred to by one eminent member of the field as: "Excellent for the medicine that was, not for the medicine that is and will be."

So much has happened so fast in the various branches of medicine and in related sciences that any priest who pursued his studies much more than ten years ago is almost hopelessly out of touch with the existing situation. Like many other areas of ethics and morality, there are far more questions than answers. Nevertheless, the ordinary priest or person connected in a professional manner with the health care profession, who needs to have some knowledge of the ethics within it, must know at least what has happened and who is saying what in order to be even remotely competent. For many years, medical ethics was a cut-and-dried field, consisting largely of approving some procedures and condemning others and then offering a rationale for the approbation or disapproval. To be sure, there have always been touchy cases and another truism has been repeated again and again: Hard cases make bad law.

Many times the priest is called upon to offer some kind of insight that will aid a physician in making a final judgment as to what course to pursue in a given case. Most clergy feel hopelessly inadequate and, if they offer answers based purely on the ethical writings of the past, they will find that their service is not very well regarded. Too much has changed too fast.

What is happening now and will almost certainly continue in the future staggers the imagination of the most sophisticated. There will be no simple answers and there will be little time to formulate answers which may prove to be critical. Perhaps this is the greatest dilemma in which the student of ethics or moral theology finds himself at the present time. Our ordinary procedure is to reflect long and deeply, consult broadly and widely and in many cases await formal pronouncement from on high before attempting to render a decision in a given case. That was a commendable way to do things and still would be if it were possible. Unfortunately, as has been noted, science, particularly medical science, proceeds at a rate far greater than the studies of ethics and morality. It is often necessary to make a decision for which there is no real precedent. There is every reason to believe that this will be more and more the case in the future. Perhaps it will come to pass that our own approach to and issuing of formal teachings will have to undergo fantastic changes in both mode and pace. In any case, the clergyman who is called upon for consultation, however infrequently, in medical matters, is going to have to be able to reason to solutions based on more than the cut-and-dried principles of the older works.

An even greater problem will be vocabulary. Both medicine and theology have changed vocabulary considerably in recent years, with the medical profession adopting one that is almost exotic. There is nothing wrong with this except that these vocabularies will change frequently and quite often will mean different things to different people. The classical vocabulary of the man in ethics or moral theology means very little to the man in the street and perhaps even less to the man in the hospital. For that reason, every effort will be made in this book to avoid all technical vocabulary on both the ethical and medical sides. Medical procedures will be explained in simple terms wherever that is possible and reference will be made to formal ethical and theological principles where that seems necessary. However, it seems quite likely that the best consultation in medical matters from a clergyman will take the form of rather plain basic speech. Further, it is almost certain he will have to base his consultation on conclusions drawn from the circumstances of each individual case. Very few universals will remain. Very few general principles will allow the kind of consultation that is really demanded.

It's worth reflecting for a moment on why the consultation is demanded in the first place. The clergyman who feels that his identity has been lost and his role changed or virtually eliminated by progress within our society may be a little surprised to find that persons in the health care professions, whatever their religious affiliation or lack of it, turn quite eagerly to the ethicist or moralist for guidance in making their own decisions. This is particularly true of those involved in the ethical or moral disciplines of the Catholic Church. The reason is simple enough. The people who consult us may not be in any particular mood to adopt our style of thinking or follow the suggestions we make, but we do have about the only consistent heritage available which they can use as a point of departure for reasoning in current cases. Catholic medical ethics and Catholic moral theology have a strong philosophical base which is lacking in almost all other sources of consultation. This is certainly a credit to those who came before us and a tribute to the worth of the Church in the modern world. However, in the consultation requested, we must offer far more than tradition even though tradition must never be neglected.

Let's answer one question right now, a question we will return to again and again as we get deeper into this book. *What is the new thrust in medical ethics?* The direction that is favored by theologians, philosophers and persons in the health care field is one of totality. Again and again we hear the phrase "total patient care."

In other words, exclusive concern with approved and forbidden procedures would be about as far out of line with the contemporary medical picture as a thing could be. The concern in the field of medical ethics now is everything that is done for and happens to a person from the moment he places himself in the hands of any person or institution to ask a question or seek to improve his health. Economics are a vital concern. So is the competence of a person performing a given procedure. Conditions in doctors' offices and clinics raise ethical questions of their own. The relationship of the patient to the administrative side of the hospital is not to be neglected. In fact, even the lowliest employee in a health care institution comes into the ethical picture. This can certainly be regarded as progress. Traditionally we have professed a great reverence for human life. However, we have rarely given much thought or much public expression to ideas concerning the quality of human life. We are going to be pressed more and more into considering quality of life as time goes on.

It cannot be overemphasized that the answers will never be simple and that even the answers indicated within this book will find many exceptions and many additional questions. There is a whole complexus of factors beyond the theoretical ethical consideration of a matter in dealing with one single patient problem. For instance, ethical thinking might suggest a particular course in treating a certain case. The doctor or hospital administrator involved in the case may very well have to ask us about the import of certain economic factors. Even where the choice appears to be rather plain, there are very often legal factors which make it necessary for a doctor or hospital to pursue the matter in a way that he himself would rather avoid. Many times he is called upon to give treatment and continue care when he knows it is pointless. However, should he strictly follow his conscience and his best medical judgment in such a matter, he may leave himself and even the institution in which he practices open to all kinds of adverse legal action. There are tensions between staff and administration and between staff, administration and trustees. There are further tensions between institutions and the community at large. All these considerations complicate decision making to the point where it is practically impossible to do anything except tackle each case by itself.

Since this book is intended primarily for parish priests, this might be a good time to explore a question that is haunting the entire Catholic health care profession at this time. It is this: Is a Catholic hospital just that, a hospital in which medicine is practiced and nursing care given in accordance with traditional Catholic teachings and presumably in a "Catholic atmosphere" or is it a community health care facility operated by Catholics who may or may not belong to a religious community or be functioning under the auspices of a Catholic diocese?

That may not sound like much of a question; in fact it's a whopper. Originally, Catholic hospitals were simply havens of charity and mercy for the sick, very often the indigent sick. Frequently they were opened in places where there were few Catholics or perhaps none. The idea was to bring the charity and mercy of Christ to those who needed it most. The nursing and the institutional tradition within the Church is something of which all of us can be proud. It goes back a very long way and has more than its share of heroes and heroines.

The picture changed somewhat as the number and influence of Catholics in the United States grew considerably, along with their ability to pay for treatment. Catholic hospitals like Catholic schools, became to a large extent places where Catholics of good faith could go for treatment assured that it would be carried out in line with the traditions and teachings of the Church. Competition for membership on Catholic hospital staffs was fierce. Rules and regulations were many and stringent. It was not at all unusual to have a sister-administrator or chaplain looking over a physician's shoulder as he pursued the science and art of medicine.

Like the schools, the hospitals grew in status and external splendor. They did inherit a certain ghetto mentality which touched all of us one way or another, but it would be quite easy to say that there was really nothing wrong with this. Patients or physicians who wished medicine practiced in a way other than that directed by the Church were free to choose other hospitals and other ways. The quality of care and training in Catholic hospitals remained quite consistently high. They were certainly nothing to be ashamed of. Many non-Catholic patients and physicians preferred them because of their excellence and general quality of care.

The world has changed swiftly. Not too many years ago it was rather a rare thing to go to the hospital. One entered it for the birth of a child, for a major operation, following an accident, or in case of some serious illness. However, as medicine expanded and improved and as new techniques became available and as different forms of financing medical care became common, the experience of being hospitalized became more and more common.

The family physician, the house call and minor surgery in the doctor's office all but disappeared from the scene, and the demand for hospital beds and increased hospital facilities grew beyond all expectations. As specialization and specialized techniques became more common, it became necessary to go to the hospital in order to have most disorders treated properly if they were at all serious.

At the same time, the population grew much faster than did the medical profession and its allied fields. Many, many people, often those with the least funds, had no place to go when suffering from minor ailments or injuries except the nearest hospital. Even expansion of out-patient care facilities and the establishment of neighborhood clinics did little to change this situation.

At the same time, just when the demand for hospital services was growing at an unprecedented rate, the number of religious sisters and brothers available to staff them stabilized, then decreased, in some cases dramatically. For the most part, one needs a very long memory to recall a nun actually nursing on a hospital floor, except as part of her training and preparation for some task to which she would be later assigned—if she remained in a religious community. In the past, many lay persons gave freely of their time and talents to Catholic hospitals, expecting little or nothing in return. Their number has decreased or remains at a level where they cannot fill all of the gaps that need to be filled.

In years past, one might choose to teach in a Catholic school or university or work in a Catholic hospital for substandard wages simply out of devotion. Such an attitude would be hard to find now and the reason is not necessarily a decline in fervor among Catholics. Much more likely, it simply reflects the terrible economic demands placed on all of us. A man or woman simply has to make a certain amount of money in order to exist. The practical effect of this has been that, in many cases, the Catholic hospital can no longer afford to open its doors to care for the indigent. Its rates generally are as high or higher than those of other hospitals. That isn't unreasonable, it faces the same costs. Nor does this mean that the indigent can or should be turned away. It simply means that the Catholic hospital administrator has to find a way to provide the same charity and mercy that Catholic hospitals have always stood for and pay the bills at the same time. This is no small task.

In the past, the gap was often taken up by private donations and endowments. These don't seem to be around as much as they were a few years ago. Even where they exist, they fall far short of meeting all of the financial needs. The result is that the Catholic hospital, like all other health care centers, must turn more and more to the community and to the Federal Government for funds in order to keep going. This presents another problem. It is axiomatic that the giver of funds usually wishes to have some say about the way in which they are used. This puts the Catholic health care facility administrator in the position of paying more and more attention to the wishes of local, state and federal governments. These wishes are often in direct conflict with the religious tradition from which he has come. Teaching and prescribing contraception and abortions on demand are only two examples of the conflicts which arise.

Like it or not, the Catholic hospital today is to most people just like any other hospital. It is a health care facility within a community to which anyone can turn in time of need. Very few administrators would wish it otherwise. Still, they are confronted by genuine problems. Should they concentrate on patients who are able and willing to pay, thereby using up beds which might be needed by those who are unable to pay? Should they bow to the wishes of various government agencies and perform certain procedures within their institutions or should they hold a hard and fast line on traditional Catholic medical ethics? To what extent are they required by their own corporate consciences to go out into the community, to provide facilities for the community? Just how binding are the norms and guidelines imposed upon them by the hierarchy? To what extent can a staff member be allowed the freedom to practice according to his own best judgment—a freedom any highly qualified physician would insist upon? The questions, in fact, are endless.

Catholic hospitals in the past have taken special pride in their obstetrical departments. These, at the present time, are threatened with extinction. The reasons are decreasing birth rates and the fact that a great many persons, including a great many Catholics, wish to have procedures performed in hospitals which are forbidden by traditional Catholic teaching. Reference is made here primarily to sterilization of females. Most physicians see nothing wrong with the performance of these procedures when requested responsibly. Most Catholic hospitals hold the line.

The result is that more and more obstetrical patients are going to non-Catholic hospitals and staff members are going more and more to other places to take care of their obstetrical patients. The OB census in many Catholic hospitals is at a dangerous low from an economic point of view. Many have closed down completely, including one just a short distance from the University of Notre Dame. Others are just getting by.

This raises far more than the question of the status of obstetrical services in Catholic hospitals. Many places require that a hospital have obstetrical facilities in order to have full accreditation. Further, obstetrical training is necessary for the hospital that wishes to have a recognized training program for interns and residents. The education of student nurses is also involved. It is hardly an answer to simply send interns and residents elsewhere for "affiliation" in order to gain their obstetrical training. The fact is, the training calls for them to learn procedures which our official guidelines state must never be performed in a Catholic hospital. Any loss of interns and residents represents a tremendous handicap to a hospital. Some Catholic hospitals are bedeviled by this loss with no real relief in sight.

Is the answer simply to relax all former disciplines and prohibitions? Many think that the line must be held. Many others see a completely different role for the Catholic health facility for the present and future. These are matters we will explore later in this book. It is only fair, though, to state at this time that the author believes, along with the great majority of persons in the field with whom he has consulted, that the role of the Catholic hospital has changed whether we like it or not. It does not stand simply as an institution to teach and enforce a certain kind of law of medical practice and a place to encourage a particular kind of religious belief. It stands, very necessarily, as an institution of service to the community at large.

This community is pluralistic in nature. It represents many dimensions and degrees of belief and opinion. The holders of these beliefs and opinions are entitled to freedom of conscience. So are physicians practicing within the existing ethical bounds of their profession. These statements are not meant to be an answer to the situation, simply a view of the situation which will be a long time in being resolved. Perhaps, as Father Richard McCormick of the Bellarmine School of Theology has said, Catholic hospitals may have to close their doors rather than "tolerate the intolerable."[1] Father McCormick is inclined to the com-

---

[1] These remarks were made during a Conference on the Ethical and Religious Directives for Health Care Facilities, held at Mercy Center, Farmington, Michigan, April 29, 1972.

munity hospital view and believes that the classical principle of toleration may often be invoked to allow a broader scope of care and policy within the Catholic hospital. Still, he realizes that cases in which a disvalue may be tolerated as the lesser of evils are not infinite and that there are practices which are truly intolerable to the Catholic conscience. The point at which he would draw the line is abortion and this point is being pressed upon us more and more.

But we have spoken here of only one small part of the total problems faced by the Catholic who has reason to reflect on ethics surrounding the health care professions and facilities. The field of genetic engineering and genetic surgery raises an endless number of questions and potential questions. At the very least, this area of concern is bound to call more and more for termination of pregnancies. It is not at all impossible that developments in this field will call for alterations in the constitution of those in fetal life. Such a course of action would have to be studied very carefully to determine its moral status.

The excessive use of drugs in everyday treatment, overly free use of elective surgery, death with dignity, death itself, rights of patients and their families, limits or the lack of them on the physician's rights to follow his own method of choice, changes in the very relationship between physician and patient . . . all of these areas will be considered in the following pages. None permits simple answers.

2. The Guidelines
and Their Critics

It is only fair, since we are addressing a primarily Catholic audience, to give full attention to the Ethical and Religious Directives for Catholic Health Care Facilities issued by the American Bishops in November 1971. Because of their length, however, we will summarize them here and publish them in full in Appendix I so that they may be referred to in their exact form according to the reader's wishes.

There was great hope in some quarters for a considerably liberalized position on the part of the hierarchy on one hand and a demand from administrators of Catholic hospitals on the other for a plain statement of its position as of now.

What resulted from the Bishops' deliberations could be described fairly as a detailed restatement of the most traditional Catholic medical ethics. Anyone who studied this field ten or even twenty years ago would find little or nothing in the document to surprise him.

Like most formal documents coming from the Church these days, some greeted the directives with enthusiasm and firm pledges of support. Others shrugged. Still others were highly critical. These latter included some of our best academic minds and their reaction could easily be described as a wail of anguish. The basic criticism is that the directives show little or no cognizance of progress in either medicine or theology. The last point is certainly not one to be taken lightly.

Even Cardinal John Dearden, who himself had approved of the directives, noted in a medical-moral symposium in April 1972[1] that there has been a fairly long history of such guidelines and that they must adjust to allow for increased knowledge of man, developments in the field of medicine and developments in our understanding of theology. There are many who would say that a new document would be called for very quickly if the Cardinal's line of reasoning is to be pursued honestly.

The most frequent criticism is that the directives are concerned entirely too much with the generative faculties and reproduction in general. After all, this represents only a small part of the total scope of medical interest. Still, whenever official pronouncements are made in the medical area, the framers of the documents seem to have an obsession with reproduction. What they have to say about it varies very little with time. This is all generally dependent on the grounds of respect, even reverence for life. Critics would be quick to comment that life involves more than embryonic and fetal life, that the quality of life provided when one is born should be considered a great deal more.

Father William Cunningham of Detroit, a man with deep and intense inner city experience says it flatly:[2] "The right to life is the right to health. There is no health where there is hunger." Sister Mary Janice Belen puts it even more directly: "Life is health."[3] In other

---

[1] Conference on the Ethical and Religious Directives for Health Care Facilities, Mercy Center, Farmington, Michigan.

[2] In a personal communication to the author.

[3] From a personal communication to the author.

words, it seems to many that there has been excessive concern with insuring conception, protecting the embryo, guarding the fetus and avoiding any deliberate termination of pregnancy except in rare cases such as a hysterectomy performed on a woman with cancer of the uterus which bears within it a non-viable fetus.

Dr. Andre Hellegers puts it rather simply: "We have to get our ethics above the umbilicus."[4] Most of the critics feel that the Bishops did little more than state the teachings of the past, with a polite nod to the present but no concession to its demands or answers to its questions. They feel that the directives have placed a kind of straightjacket on a Catholic health care facility that desires to be completely faithful to the directives of the Church.

Little is said about the community at large in the directives and many critics feel that the hospital, like the parish, is responsible for anyone within its area, not simply those who hold to strictly orthodox traditional Catholic views. They particularly dislike the section that makes the teachings of the Bishops binding on all staff and on all personnel within the Catholic health care facility whatever their private convictions may be. They feel that the whole concept of religious liberty is considerably endangered by the hierarchical stance. This may not seem like much of a point, but the fact is that in many places, especially inner city areas, the Catholic hospital may be the major employer. Many of the critics feel that it is quite possible for the Catholic hospital to retain its identity and its integrity while becoming more and more an institution that serves the general public and respects the legitimate views and

---

[4] Conference on the Ethical and Religious Directives for Health Care Facilities, Mercy Center, Farmington, Michigan, April 1972.

conscience of that public and the physicians who serve it. About the only area where there is consistent resistance is abortion.

But where does this leave the teaching Church? Father McCormick, quoted before, is one critic who sees no real problem. He says that the imposed decision, so common in the past, will be increasingly hard to enforce and that its enforcement becomes less and less desirable in a pluralistic community. He believes that it is possible to believe and to hold certain standards without insisting that these standards be observed at all times by all persons who do not share the beliefs.

Furthermore, he sees reflective dissent from magisterial teachings as "the beginning of new evidence." He remarks that the authority to teach is not the authority to decide. "The teaching-learning process is involved and it is more important than obedience," he says. "One does not obey teachers."[5]

Dr. Warren Reich states the matter somewhat differently. He says that non-infallible papal teaching, properly understood, is not a divine norm, is not revelation and must have a "characteristic of tentativeness."[6] One might add that it is unfair to the magisterium itself to ask it to come up with answers for questions which have not yet been raised. The coming of new knowledge is bound to raise questions which the most serious curial theologian could not possibly anticipate.

The critics also cite the problems that exist in Catholic hospitals which may be the only health care facilities in their communities. Their response to the directives may be viewed a little differently because of

[5] *Ibid.*
[6] *Ibid.*

the limits on their options. That's looking at it a little academically. In practice what often happens is that a physician who practices in a Catholic hospital which is the only one in a given community simply moves patients desiring certain procedures (such as sterilization) to health care facilities outside the community. This is a weaseling sort of answer, but the kind found most frequently in our society and it certainly is not an answer that settles the basic question.

Again and again the Catholic physicians and Catholic health care facilities as well as the teachers on whom they depend have been accused of imposing undue hardship and even agony on persons who go to them in good conscience when they withhold certain treatment in order to hold the line on tradition. Few would hold that any deliberate cruelty is intended. In truth, though, many cases of suffering could be noted. Still, the traditionalist will insist that adhering to authentic moral teachings does involve a certain amount of pain and inconvenience on many occasions and that there is simply no way of escaping this. In all fairness it should be stated here again that a good many reputable moralists feel that the directives offered by the Bishops express doctrine, that they do teach, and that the hospital teaches the community by insisting upon them and enforcing them.

In no sense is the situation an easy one for anyone concerned. As previously noted, hard cases make bad law, but it is worth reporting just a few of the things that have happened in recent years to illustrate the nature of the difficulties faced by Catholic health care facilities.

There is a hospital in Alaska which is owned and operated by the county but administered and largely staffed by members of a religious community. An abortion on demand law was passed. In all truth, the options open to the religious were very limited indeed.

Dr. Hellegers reports a case at Georgetown where an extremely obese mother of ten was admitted because of special equipment which would enable physicians to determine the age of the fetus in a woman of her structure. Upon admission she expressed a wish for tubal ligation. She was told that this would not be possible at Georgetown. She decided that she would have her baby, delivered vaginally as in the past, and then go to another hospital for the sterilization operation.

However, she developed pre-eclampsia, a toxic condition of the uterus, which was complicated by a critically irregular fetal heart beat. A cesarean section was indicated. She requested that a tubal ligation be performed at the time of the section. She was told that this would not be possible at Georgetown. It is a sterilization procedure, "tube tying."

The mother complained that she felt it was unfair to have abdominal surgery twice in a period of less than two months to satisfy the policies of a given hospital. The matter was discussed at length and finally solved by transferring her to another facility where the baby was delivered by cesarean section and the tubal ligation performed.

Dr. Hellegers notes that there was a distinct risk of fetal death in transit to the other hospital. Had that occurred, Georgetown might well have been open to a malpractice suit. Dr. Hellegers confesses that he had grave moral problems with the entire case and comments: "Had it come to court I would have had to testify that there was malpractice, perhaps morally justified, but still malpractice."[7]

---

[7] *Ibid.*

By way of general information, malpractice is considered to be failure to perform those procedures which are considered normal, acceptable medical practice in the community.

About the same time Georgetown found itself in another unusual position in that it turned down a large and badly needed research grant because the research involved would have required obtaining semen samples by means of masturbation. Prohibition of obtaining samples by this means, traditionally forbidden by the Church, is considered little more than silly by many people in both the medical and theological professions and there was some hope that it would come up for discussion prior to the issuing of the Bishops' Directives printed here. As one physician noted when the Directives were issued without any change in position: "Well it didn't come up this time. Masturbation will just have to wait until next year."

Another example of the effects of what many consider to be overly restrictive policies emanating from the Church involves research into a medication which would regulate rather than suspend ovulation. For all practical purposes, such a medication would end most of the controversy over contraception. However, certain physicians who have appeared before government hearings in an effort to obtain research funds to develop this medication have been severely criticized by the hierarchy because the government hearings involved were concerned with population control, a word which is just plain verboten in the upper spheres of Church government. In this instance, the criticism may well have kept some doctors from testifying and that, in turn, may have prevented or limited research grants which would have led to developments which would have been very much to the Church's benefit.

There is another way in which the stringent policies of the Church, interpreted with extreme strictness has worked against what many consider to be the best interests of the Church and its members. Doctor John Doran, a Detroit OB-GYN man, said in a recent address that an important opportunity for counseling has been lost because people under thirty generally give no consideration whatever to the morality or immorality of contraception and sterilization. He says that he has found this to be the case in his own practice, that his findings are echoed by others in his specialty and that their experience is similar to that of confessors.[8]

What it all comes down to is this. The Church has never flatly condemned limiting the size of one's family. The traditional teachings were that for a reason of sufficient weight, parents could decide to limit the number of their children, provided that they did this either by abstaining from intercourse or practicing the rhythm method. One of the things that priests were taught to caution such parents about was undertaking the limitation of family size purely on selfish grounds. Legitimate use of the rhythm system or even abstaining from sex purely for the purpose of avoiding further children was seen to be a disvalue if done for anything less than good and weighty reasons such as economic hardship or hardship of health to either one of the parties. Refusing to have children simply to maintain a very high standard of living or to avoid the inconvenience of having children or anything else that smacked of selfishness was not considered to be a just cause for family limitation.

Long before *Humanae Vitae* was promulgated, a

---

[8] *Ibid.*

great many Catholic couples had already decided the matter of contraception for themselves. The Church had taken too long to express itself on a question that was too pressing to allow for indefinite waiting. Just as it is true in much of the history of theology of marriage, the actual solutions came out of life as it was lived, not from the document *Humanae Vitae*.

A great many theologians and physicians for that matter find many weaknesses in the document which is the authentic teaching of the Church. However, that is not the point. People waited as long as they could wait and then formed their own consciences on the matter. Younger people thought the whole argument was pretty silly and made up their minds to go ahead with contraception regardless of the teachings of the document. In so doing, they eliminated the possibility of serious discussion of reasons for family planning with physicians and priests. It is felt by many pastors that in this respect *Humanae Vitae* actually led to a certain amount of immorality; many couples are now arranging to remain childless for various periods of time for reasons which would not be considered of sufficient weight if one viewed the situation in its full moral context. Time and again, we seem to have defeated ourselves by our own unwillingness to bend to the realities of life. Whether or not this is justified by the position of the magisterium is not for me to settle here. The cases I note, however, are very real and should not be passed over lightly.

The point seems to pop up again and again and again. Because of our own rigidity and our own traditional unwillingness to alter traditional paths, we have often weakened our own general position, lost things that we needed badly and perhaps even encouraged immorality in the name of enforcing morality. In the practical order there are quite a few cases on record where Catholic hospitals have lost badly needed government funds because of a lack of lay membership representative of the community on the board of trustees. I know of three such cases in Detroit within the last year. It would seem that if we are going to operate community health care facilities, we are going to have to listen to the community and extend to the community its full rights, even when this involves accepting ideas with which we do not fully agree.

The whole matter is far too involved to be settled here. The only reason for presenting it in such detail is to give some idea of the complexity of ethical problems faced by Catholic physicians and Catholic health care facilities today as opposed to those of say twenty years ago when there was an argument over the licitness of having a non-Catholic clergyman attend a dying non-Catholic patient in a Catholic hospital.

It seems very likely the ordinary priest called upon for consultation in medical matters is going to have to exercise a kind of pastoral judgment, a judgment which consists of considerable latitude in making up his mind. This has long been the case in other matters, such as handling various kinds of marriage cases. A rule of thumb, far less than a dogmatic teaching but very useful in practice, is that a good human solution is quite often the best Christian solution.

Author's Note: For further discussion, see "The Present Status of the Ethical and Religious Directives for Catholic Health Facilities" by Rev. Anthony R. Kosnik, *Linacre Quarterly,* May 1973.

3. Contraception, Sterilization and Abortion

As noted earlier, a great many of the faithful have already made up their minds on the morality of contraception and sterilization. Moreover, little if anything can be expected in the way of further formal teaching on these subjects. The whole situation is lamentable in that a great many careless and sometimes purely selfish uses are being made of contraception and sterilization. Many people, not excluding all clergy, simply threw up their hands at the way the official Church has approached these matters. In throwing up their hands, they stopped devoting any particularly deep thought prior to making decisions. Certainly this was not the intent of the Church teachers.

It comes down to a couple of very interesting points. One was passed over almost casually by Dr. Warren Reich, during a recent medical-moral symposium. He said: "Man has complete dominion over his body, including his generative faculties."[1]

---

[1] Conference on the Ethical and Religious Directives for Health Care Facilities, Mercy Center, Farmington, Michigan, April 1972.

I was somewhat surprised that no one jumped to his feet to challenge that statement, since many older moral authors have made it very plain that man does not have complete dominion over his body—that it is, in effect, lent to him by God during his days on earth and is to be used according to the will of God insofar as is known to the individual. This view, then, led to an attitude whereby Church teachings, whatever their real status in authenticity and infallibility might be, were passed on as the will of God in the field of medical ethics. A patient was simply told that such and such a thing could not be done because it was forbidden by the Church. If the man took seriously the total dominion of God over his body and also took seriously the Church as the one invariably certain spokesman of God's will, he usually went along with the restrictions or prohibitions whatever they were.

The point itself could be argued endlessly. Since God made man, the world and all that is in it, he could certainly be said to have dominion over them. By the same token, as early as Genesis, he gives dominion to man. As for total dominion of man over his own body, the fact is that he can exercise it whether the Church approves or not. It might be said that he exercises his dominion in an immoral manner, but the fact remains that each individual can exert a virtually complete dominion over his body, subject to its own limitations and the circumstances under which he lives. For all practical purposes then, the old notion of God lending man his body to use according to the will of God seems to be less desirable in the present day than the notion that man himself has total dominion and must consider how this power may be exercised in the most moral manner.

As already noted, Catholic physicians and theologians have to a great extent liberalized their views on contraception and sterilization. With few exceptions this cannot be said about abortion. An example of positions held rather widely by serious and competent physicians and theologians is this statement:

A PROPOSED RECOMMENDATION FOR STERILIZATION POLICY IN CATHOLIC HEALTH CARE INSTITUTIONS

Summary of consensus opinions reached at a meeting on October 18, 1971 at Wayne County Society Headquarters with the chairmen of the obstetrical departments of Catholic hospitals in the Archdiocese of Detroit, the Medical Morals Committee of the Catholic Physicians' Guild of Detroit and Fr. Anthony Kosnik, theological consultant.

I. Surgical sterilization allowed as outlined below with the approval of the Chairman of the Obstetrical Department of the hospital in which the operation is to be done or his designate (committee or consultant)

   A. fetal indications
   1. past history of severe erythroblastosis
   2. predictable inheritable defect of a serious nature such as Tay-Sachs disease, phenylketonuria
   B. maternal indications
   1. conditions that would be directly affected by a subsequent pregnancy and delivery such as a serious cardiovascular or renal disease, diabetes or a weakened uterine scar or pelvic adhesions

    2. conditions rendering mothering and child care difficult or improbable because of serious illness such as a malignant disorder, serious neurological or neuro-muscular disorder or connective tissue disease such as rheumatoid arthritis or lupus erythenatosis

II. cases not included in the above categories in which a department chairman feels sterilization appropriate should be presented to the Archdiocesan Medical Morals Committee for approval prior to surgery

III. case reports of all patients sterilized will be filed with the Archdiocesan Medical Morals Committee for a review on a monthly basis

IV. upon assurance that the patient is aware of the moral considerations and with due respect for personal convictions, non-abortifacient family planning methods should be appropriately taught and prescribed in the out-patient clinics of the above hospitals.[2]

Of course, this could not be called official Church teaching or policy in any sense, but since it represents the thinking of a sizable number of very responsible Catholics, it is hard to ignore. If personal experience and wide conversation are worth anything at all as criteria, the material presented in this document is not foreïgn in Catholic circles today. In fact, some physicians and moralists would go beyond what is included in the statement. Some are inclined to approve steriliza-

---

[2] See also *Policy Manual for Committee to Advise on Requests for Obstetrical/Gynaecological Sterilization Procedures*, St. Joseph's Hospital, London, Ontario.

tion for schizophrenics because of the possibility of inheritance of that disorder and also because of the particular agony suffered by schizophrenic mothers during pregnancy and birth. The same could be said about those who are irreversibly mentally retarded.

What is happening is the extension of a tendency which has become more and more common in recent years to lean toward the person rather than the institution in making critical ethical decisions. There has long been a tendency in the hierarchy to defend certain principles to the death rather than admit that things once stated in a rather universal manner may have been in error or may have been enforced too rigidly. It is sad to say that those in power have frequently been able to tolerate considerable human suffering rather than compromise even one minute teaching. On the official level, the juridical mind prevails. The preamble of the Bishops' Directives quoted in Appendix I certainly reflects a juridical mind and a kind of ecclesiology which might be called a little bit less than contemporary. Originally, a preamble was submitted by a number of theologians who sought to have the tenor of the Bishops' statement more oriented to the realities of the present and the possibilities of the future. The suggested preamble was rejected in favor of the one which we have.

Many moralists as well as physicians would be even freer than the statement presented here indicates if it were possible to recommend reversible sterilization. At the present time, there are no procedures guaranteed to be reversible. In the case of vasectomy, sterilization of the male, attempts to reverse the procedure have met relatively limited success. It is not at all impossible, however, that reversible sterilization will be a matter of course before too long. This would certainly open the door to even broader views.

As for abortion, there is a great deal of discussion and a great deal of deep study along with a great deal of argument, but it is safe to say that a large consensus of the Catholic medical-moral community still opposes direct termination of pregnancy. Matters involved in the principle of the two-fold effect, such as a cancerous uterus, or a positively diagnosed ectopic pregnancy (pregnancy in the fallopian tube) are treated quite leniently, but these cases do not allow us to reason to any freer position in the matter of directly intended termination of pregnancy simply for the general welfare of the mother or because of her particular wishes. There are a number of physicians, including Dr. Hellegers, who state rather flatly that abortion in general is medically contraindicated.[3]

In the matter of ectopic pregnancies the usual and approved surgical procedure once a positive diagnosis is obtained is to remove the tube in which the pregnancy exists. In this, there is no conflict with traditional Catholic medical ethics. A more recent procedure is a delicate one in which the fetus is scraped from the tube, thereby preserving the tube intact. Traditional Catholic moralists have opposed this as direct abortion. A number of other moral thinkers within Catholic circles regard this prohibition as silly because the fetus has no chance of attaining full human life and the procedure results in keeping the female reproductive organs intact.

We have reports from Japan, England and other places which indicate that free and easy abortion is not the panacea that was hoped for. Still, there is a great

---

[3] At the Farmington Conference.

pressure in society for greatly liberalized abortion laws and policies. Many thinkers that I know within the Church feel that there is no particular reason for us to go to any great length to strengthen or maintain existing laws prohibiting abortions. This is simply a matter of saying that, while they don't approve of abortions themselves, they do not feel that they have an obligation to cause and enforce civil law prohibiting them.

This is an instance where many women do claim total dominion of their total bodies and are not going to split hairs to the extent of considering that in having an abortion they are dealing with more than their own bodies. In any case abortions are extremely common and will probably become more common and there is little solace in the fact that they are generally being performed under more sanitary conditions and by more competent personnel. In no case can this be written off easily as the lesser of evils. Official Catholic position on abortion is not likely to change in the near future or ever. There is, however, a growing disposition to stop fighting for particular anti-abortion laws, without allowing for any compromise in our own position.

It is surprising to me, however, to find a rather substantial number of Catholics who find nothing at all wrong with abortion. I've even argued the point with nuns. Generally, they will cite exceptional cases and cases which appealed to sentiment as well as one's own best human instincts. They will ask you: "OK that's what you say as a theologian. What do you really say as a man? What would you the man do confronted with such a case?"

To their dismay I have held very firmly that I could never, at least as I see things now, condone deliberate direct termination of normal pregnancy unless the case involved a clear-cut application of the principle of the two-fold effect and met all of its requirements perfectly. That's virtually impossible in direct termination.

The case most often thrown at the Catholic moralist, and I'm quite sure at the ordinary priest, is the case of rape in which a totally innocent person is faced with an unwanted and I suppose we could say without quibbling an unjust pregnancy. Dr. Reich is one theologian who believes that in the case of rape the rights of the victim have been violated and she therefore has no duty to continue the pregnancy.[4] This would have to be classed as a minority viewpoint. However, more and more Catholic doctors are voicing approval of abortion in various forms. They do not represent a uniform voice, but the greatest problem is that in practice they may be performing abortions and using rather poor reasoning to justify the action.

One such case was that of a Michigan OB-GYN man, a devout Catholic, intensely interested in good medical ethics, who asked me if I believed in capital punishment. I answered no. He asked me if I believed in the just war. Again I answered no. He asked me if I believed in self defense. Not being a totally non-violent person, I answered that I did and he was quick to tell me that confronted in a dark alley by an aggressor I would probably blow his brains out. To be perfectly honest, he is probably right. I asked him what this had to do with abortion and he replied: "Sometimes you have to kill."

As far as he was concerned, where there was an unwanted pregnancy and a sufficiently strong human motivation to terminate it, abortion was allowable. He

[4] *Ibid.*

cited cases of pregnancy involving uninformed teen-agers and pregnancies resulting from intercourse be-tween retardates and said that the pregnancies were the result of acts which "were not human acts." I don't find his reasoning very compelling. In fact, it suggests a kind of punitive morality, with pregnancy as the punishment for a fully immoral action of sexual in-tercourse. Insofar as I can set the situation straight in my own mind, pregnancy never should be viewed as punishment, simply as a result of an action whether it be a fully human act or not. Terminating a pregnancy because the pregnant girl does not deserve punishment, is hardly a compelling reason for advocating abortion in my mind.

As I said, the rape case is the one that will be thrown at you most often in day-to-day operation. Its classic form is this: "Suppose my 15-year-old daughter is on her way home tonight and is raped. Do you mean to say there is nothing at all that you can do?"

If by that is meant is there no way that I can weasel around and come up with a justification for abortion, my answer would have to be no, there is nothing I can do. A number of evasions and rationalizations might be applied in a case like this, but to invoke them would be to deny the kind of morality I have been trying to build up over the years, one which is not legalistic in nature and which does not seek to circumvent law, one which is in fact above the letter of the law and in the spirit of the law, urging upon all persons an honest quest for perfection. To become a moral or medical shyster in such case, seems to me to be selling out completely.

However, some very wise authorities on the subject point out that in such a case we are dealing with probabilities. The probability of the girl being made pregnant by rape is likely to be low. Present-day procedures make it possible to determine with a high degree of accuracy whether or not conception has occurred within 48 hours of the actual intercourse.

There appears to be one way out in such cases which is considered tolerable by some very good Catholic people, although I am sure a great number would oppose it. If, following an attack and rape, the victim is taken to the hospital as an emergency patient, the normal procedure consists of a certain amount of washing and cleansing of the female organs. In fact, this is necessary in order to obtain a semen sample which could be used to establish legally that rape had occurred and which might prove to be essential evidence in prosecution of the rapist. In a case like this, where "washing out" is pretty routine procedure, I know many Catholic physicians and administrators who would not hesitate to say: "Wash away and wash away thoroughly." Particular attention is paid to the tubes, because it is most likely that a thorough cleansing of the tubes would be the best preventive measure insofar as pregnancy is concerned. One very conservative GYN man has even suggested the use of certain medications to flood the tubes under such circumstances.

Here we come down to a good deal of hair splitting. Are we actually talking about terminating pregnancy or are we merely talking about a kind of vigorous contraception? Since we have no way of knowing in these emergency circumstances if conception has yet occurred, chances are it has not.

To be sure, this is an extreme case, calling for a particular set of circumstances and even then there is not a great deal of agreement on the procedure of choice or the extent to which it should be carried out. The range of opinion goes all the way from minimal interference with the possibility of conception to the attitude of "scrape away and be damned."

I hate to keep coming back to it, but this is another classic example of the cliche, "Hard cases make bad law." We can draw very few conclusions from this controversy that would have any particular effect on other matters pertaining to abortion. We have long since given up arguing at what point the soul is "infused" in the body and there is no great certainty as to when a fertilized ovum becomes a human in development. The argument against abortion used by most modern moralists is based on the potential of human life and the necessity of protecting that rather than on any attempt to decide when human life actually originates. Others say that a fertilized ovum is biologically complete, human.

Discussion is bound to increase involving the so-called "morning after pills" which may take various forms involving various physiological actions. The pills stand a strong chance of great popularity if expense and frequent severe side-effects are not involved.

The ethical problem here is interesting if not clear-cut. Conception needn't have occurred between coitus and the "morning after." On the other hand, conception may have occurred or may be so close to highly probable occurrence that the pill, if effective, would have to be considered an abortifacient. Granted, the taker would never know, but it is difficult to see easy justification of these medications, especially since they often avoid the careful consideration for family limitation presumably involved in responsible contraception by those at all concerned with Catholic morality, even though they are at odds with the Pope's teaching. The procreative act has occurred.

Apparently the "morning after pills" make a favorable opinion next to impossible and even their use in "unjust aggressor" cases such as rape would be difficult to live with because of the abortifacient possibility. I am sure there are opinions widely varying from this in some liberal circles, including Catholic ones.[5]

As the procedure called amniocentisis—study of the amniotic fluid which surrounds the fetus *in utero*—continues to develop, there will probably be more and more pressure for abortions. Medical personnel are able to learn quite a bit about the fetus from the study of this fluid, obtained from a tap of the mother's abdomen. It is possible to spot a defective child in development. To date, the most general use of the information obtained from amniocentisis is in a case of fetuses suffering as a result of RH factors. It is possible to give the fetus a transfusion *in utero* which may do a great deal to solve the whole problem. Similarly, treatments will probably come along which will allow corrections of certain conditions or defects in the fetus before birth occurs. So long as these are aimed at improving the health and general condition of the fetus and involve no particular risk to either fetus or mother, there is little than can be said against them.

However, there is almost certain to be great pressure for the destruction of fetuses which are found to be irreversibly defective. It is quite likely that many mothers, provided with this kind of information, would

---

[5] This assumes there will in time be various "morning after pills." The present medication, Diethylstilbestrol (DES), is hazardous because if a pregnancy persists, there is high probability of vaginal cancer in a female offspring.

be inclined to favor termination of the pregnancy. So would a great many medical men. But, strictly from the standpoint of ethics and morality, abortion is abortion, whether it is performed in the name of preserving the mother's mental health or whether it is to prevent the birth of a defective child.

Where amniocentisis shows high probability that a defective fetus exists, there are Catholic moralists who see nothing wrong with direct abortion. For instance, in a case with the XXY chromosome, associated with criminal behavior, notably sexual criminal behavior, even a leading German moralist has said he would not oppose direct termination of the pregnancy by means of abortion.[6] However, this whole business is still the subject of a great deal of argument and few are particularly willing to say that the official Church teaching should be changed in any way. What is being urged is that certain specific cases might allow for direct intended termination of a pregnancy and that surgical procedures would be undertaken only after exhaustive study and consultation. It is unlikely that any official change will be forthcoming for a very long time.

Good genetic counseling, another whole area of study, could do a great deal to prevent the conception of defective children and it would seem to many that this is a much healthier direction for us to follow than one which leads us to any increased tolerance of direct intended termination of pregnancy.

A great many defectives are born every year and they in turn carry with them the threat of producing still more defectives. This is a tragedy and it is certainly a condition that any medical man or any moralist would like to do something about. It would seem,

---

[6] During a private conversation among theologians.

though, that officially we are rather firmly locked in a traditional position. The end does not justify the means.

The working priest is going to have a terrible time dealing with cases such as we have touched on here. There have been tremendous changes in community attitudes, and that certainly includes the attitude of Catholics within the community. Whereas we have said traditionally that the purpose of sex is the procreation and education of children along with fulfillment of married love, the general attitude in society today (and I believe this includes a large segment of Catholic society) is that the purpose of sex is sex. For all practical purposes, the sex act has been separated from any view of its being primarily or essentially a reproductive action. It is seen as an expression of love, as a relief of tensions, as a legitimate source of fun and enjoyment. It is impossible to argue completely with these things, but surely the procreative aspects of sex cannot simply be written off because of a change in community disposition.

The science of genetics and the possibilities that it will present to us in the near future may do a great deal to solve some of the problems we have been talking about here. At the same time, a great many within the genetics field have a rather fascistic utopian view of their work. They see the possibility of man controlling not only the quantity but the quality of mankind. It is very hard to escape the notion that this comes very close to playing God.

If the ultimate choices as to who shall not have children and who shall and when they shall have them and what will happen when things go wrong genetically are left in the hands of an elitist group of physicians and other scientists, we may have a situation on our hands much worse than any that can be fostered by the very worst of curial theologians.

At the present time it is simply much too early to try to set policies and principles in this whole matter, but one needs to be aware of the potential. It does seem entirely possible that a reasonable, entirely moral solution to the whole thing can evolve if we are careful enough to keep abreast of developing fields within science, think through our own positions thoroughly and communicate them plainly and constantly.

To be sure, there are real problems. Medical science has kept more people alive longer. This has had a direct result on the genetic problems we face. Many persons who would have died without reproducing are alive and reproducing. In general that would seem to be something to rejoice about, but it does present problems. People possessing inheritable disorders, such as diabetes, are staying around this earth longer and turning out more diabetics. An extremist view is that we will have a population comprised of a fearful number of diabetics before very long. In addition to that, it is estimated that twenty percent of the existing population carries some deleterious mutation, that is the possibility of reproducing a really troublesome defective. If these in turn propagate readily, the future of our race is not to be seen as an especially happy one, where we had assumed that things were getting better and better because we were able to do more and more to keep people healthier and to keep them alive longer.

Genetics certainly is going to have something to say on the matter, although at present most of what is said is in the speculative stage and no hard and fast positions are possible for us. There is, however, nothing wrong with giving serious consideration to the views of Dr. Tommy Evans of Wayne State University who feels that we are paying much too much attention to population problems and insufficient attention to the quality of reproduction.[7]

However that may be, it is difficult to predict that the Catholic Church as an institution will change very much in its view of abortion. It is difficult to see anything wrong with seeking genetic counseling prior to marriage and one may even argue that there is a definite obligation to avoid a marriage, the offspring of which are in all probability going to become problems. Genetic counseling after marriage, should it present a negative picture, leads to questions of sterilization and contraception. As has been noted, the general view of sterilization and contraception has been liberalized to quite an extent in the general population and the actual practice of medicine if not in the official teaching of the Church.

---

[7] "Too Many Defective Human Beings," *Detroit Free Press*, July 23, 1972.

4. Life and Death

Once, within my own lifetime, the determination of life and death was a fairly simple matter, although never one without problems.

The development of various machines and techniques of prolonging the life of the seriously ill has forced us to take a new look at the whole situation. The development of transplant surgery has raised serious questions as to when a man or woman is really dead. As is true in almost all areas of medical practice today, the answers do not come easily or readily and the answers may not last for too long.

Dr. Elisabeth Kubler-Ross, in her book, *On Death and Dying,* has made a profound contribution to the field by pointing out how much our fear of dying influences the way that we care for the living, especially those of the living who may be approaching death. She even sees fault on the part of medical and hospital personnel who will do almost anything rather than admit that a patient is dying and may delay for an unreasonable length of time informing him and his family of the true situation. This is probably neither good medicine nor good ethics.

Let's state a few things clearly. Death is a fact which each of us has to face. Sometimes it comes in sudden, senseless almost perverse forms. Other times it comes over a period of time so extended as to seem unreasonably cruel. But one way or another, it comes to us all. Knowing this and facing this is every bit as important as knowing that one will have a birthday next year, if he lives, or that one will undergo certain physiological changes as he ages.

It is indeed a pitiful thing to see a child die. It's a sad thing to see a young parent die. Nevertheless, these things will occur and for each one of us death is an absolute certainty. So is disintegration of the human body after death, even though the material of the body remains in the earth and eventually becomes part of it.

As Christians, we have been assured by God himself, speaking through scripture and the Church, that man has an immortal soul and that his body will rise at the end of time. Just how that is to be accomplished remains the subject of a great deal of pious speculation and accounts for the needless creation of stories. God has promised us these things, the Church has guaranteed them dogmatically. If we ask any more, perhaps we might question the depth and intensity of our own faith.

Unfortunately, certain platonic and neoplatonic notions of the soul have led us to construct various systems of thought to explain life after biological death. Deep within all of us there is the idea of a huge number of disembodied souls floating around in some form of happiness in a place called heaven. This is not meant irreverently, it is simply to say that the Church has never been specific and cannot be very specific on the precise manner in which the soul's immortality is lived out. Neither can it explain with anything more than the eyes and voice of faith how a disintegrated body can be brought to life at the time of the general resurrection. These are things we know through faith and most of us would be a lot better off if they had been passed on to us in this simple form.

We can contribute at least a little something by making sure that the children we teach either as parents or teachers do not get superstitious, magical or cartoon-like notions of heaven and the afterlife. Man lives after death because God says so. Man will rise because God promised this. Beyond this, we know very little. What more can you ask?

Knowing these things it is somewhat surprising that we maintain a deep and terrible fear of death. The only answer is that we do not take the promises of God seriously enough. If we did, death would hold no particular terror for us even though no one looks forward to suffering and leaving behind the things of his lifetime: his family, his friends, all of his belongings and earthly pursuits. It is this very notion that leads us to a theological solution which may be of some help within the realm of medical ethics, where the whole question of life and death is still very much controverted.

Recently, Father Anthony Kosnik was called to a hospital to speak to nurses who were greatly disturbed that organs were being removed from patients in order to be used as transplants. The donor patients' hearts were still beating. By all of our old-time standards, these people were still alive and were perhaps "murdered" in order to effect transplant surgery.

Father Kosnik, a moderate and thoughtful man, reassured them in the following manner: "Life is relational. Theological death occurs with the permanent, irreversible, decisive, definitive orientation of relational activity."[1]

---

[1] Direct communication to the author.

In other words a person who cannot relate to the people and things around him and for whom there is no hope of restoration of relational activity, is considered to be dead. Therefore, the fact that his heart might be still beating raises no particular moral question.

Looking at it another way, we are in the habit of thinking of "the moment of death" or worse yet, the moment when the soul leaves the body. Practically speaking, one does not die in a moment, but in a series of degrees. Death is a process. The precise point when one can be said to be dead is not one on which there is consistant agreement among medical, legal and religious scholars. For a long time it was sufficient to determine that the heart had stopped beating, that there was no respiration taking place and that the patient lacked any reflexes at all. To be sure there were some hasty and accidental pronouncements of death along the way, but anyone who has been around the dead and the dying for any length of time has little practical difficulty in deciding when a person is dead.

The problem comes largely from the fact that life can be sustained, even in a person whose relational activity has ceased and cannot possibly return, by use of respirators and other involved, sometimes exotic means. A patient who could be described as an "unburied corpse" can be kept breathing and his heart can be kept beating for a long, long period by mechanical means. Among other things, this led to consideration of the use of the electroencephalogram to determine when brain life ceased. All too many writers, including some who have published in otherwise responsible Church journals, have said that we now determine death by the cessation of brain waves. That is not exactly the case.

From a clinical point of view, to be absolutely certain that death has occurred we would have to have determination that cardiac, pulmonary and brain activity had ceased and that the heart and pulmonary activity could not be continued without artificial, mechanical support. Actually scientists have been able to keep human specimens "alive" for great periods of time. Cells do not die easily if they are given assistance in living. However, here we are talking about biological matters, not the actual death of a human person.

As for the transplant/donor situation, it has become obvious that a number of serious restraints, which may take the form of law before long, must be observed. A "clinical death" such as described above, should be demanded before any procedures are performed on the patient for the purpose of obtaining one or more organs for transplant purposes. Since those involved in the transplant surgery have an understandable wish to get the donor organs as soon as possible, it is general practice to exclude them from the group which decides upon the death of the donor. A further principle should be that there should be no real difference in consideration in the death of a non-donor and the death of a donor. For all practical purposes a person should be dead before an organ can be removed for transplant, except in cases where a donor may give an organ without any real question of losing his life in the process.

None of this is going to be terribly easy. Father Kosnik's concept of theological death puts theologically trained persons at ease and may make it possible for them to offer wiser and more prudent counsel to families of the dying and to medical personnel. The fact remains, however, that a doctor must be terribly careful before stating with certainty that a patient is dead. He faces vast, perhaps ruinous consequences if he does anything other than exercise every possible precaution against premature pronouncement of death.

An old notion that is still very much with us is that everything should be done to preserve life until it is certain that it can no longer be preserved. This has led to the employment of an unbelievable assortment of artificial means for maintaining a kind of biological life in patients whom Father Kosnik would say are certainly dead. Many doctors feel called upon according to the best lights of their consciences to employ any and every means to preserve any semblance of life in a patient. Others could be said to be a bit too casual in deciding that there isn't much point in extending ordinary measures to preserve a life that can never be a fully human one again.

An exact answer to this is impossible, and it is important that the priest realizes this as he is approached for consultation either by family or by physician. Actually, we can rely here on some very old principles which were stated with great clarity by Pope Pius XII. Man has a moral obligation to use ordinary means to preserve life and health. There is no obligation to employ extraordinary means. Gerald Kelly, S.J., puts it this way:

> *Ordinary* means of preserving life are all medicines, treatments and operations which offer a reasonable hope of benefit for the patient and which can be obtained and used without excessive expense, pain or other inconvenience. *Extraordinary* means of preserving life means all medicines, treatments and operations which cannot be obtained and used without excessive expense,

pain or other inconvenience or if used would not offer a reasonable hope of benefit. . . . one may but need not use extraordinary means to preserve life.[2]

Edwin Healy, S.J., says:

> We may define as an extraordinary means whatever cure now is very costly, or very unusual or very painful or very difficult or very dangerous or if the good effects that can be expected from its use are not proportionate to the difficulty or inconvenience that are entailed.[3]

In other words, we are left with very few hard and fast approaches to answers as to how long a patient should be kept alive by heroic artificial means. It is certainly not ordinarily immoral to make a maximum effort to preserve and prolong life, but neither is it necessary. One great complicating factor of which we have become increasingly aware in recent years is the fact that more and more it is difficult to say which means are ordinary and which are extraordinary. Administration of oxygen, cardiac stimulants and similar treatment would be considered almost always by almost everyone as ordinary. However, use of recent developments in life prolonging procedures is so common that some persons would certainly hold that they constitute ordinary means. Things we haven't yet dreamed of will become in time extraordinary means and then so common as to raise the question as to whether they are ordinary.

---

[2] *Medico-Moral Problems* (St. Louis, Mo.: The Catholic Hospital Assn., 1958), p. 129.

[3] *Medical Ethics* (Chicago: Loyola University Press, 1956), p. 67.

In any case, complex judgments which will not allow a rubber stamp of approval on the head of him making the judgment, are the order of the day. One way we can get around the problem of the extraordinary becoming the ordinary is to make a distinction between customary and ordinary. A means may be customary in that it is quite common and is usually applied. It may still qualify as extraordinary if it involves extended pain and suffering, grave expense, grave inconvenience and little or no hope of effecting anything like a cure. The more that the patient approaches Father Kosnik's criterion for theological death, the more this could be said to be the case.

It should be added that there are conditions under which even ordinary means are not required. A couple of classical examples are the case of a man about to be burned to death by his enemies. He has available to him several buckets of water. Water is certainly an ordinary means of putting out fire, but if using the water to put out fire would only prolong the agony of burning to death, it is held that the man has no obligation to make use of the buckets. Another old chestnut is the case of a man who is given some food when he is in the process of starvation. He would be using ordinary means by consuming the food, but if he has no real guarantee that there will be more food and that the food that he has received will only prolong the agony of starvation, he has no obligation to eat.

The patient's own choice is a thing that is frequently neglected. Many patients express clear-cut wishes to be spared long, lingering death processes as vegetables. However, their families frequently feel that they are acting immorally unless they prolong the process as far as possible. In this, they are often encouraged by physicians, some of whom honestly believe that they have an obligation in ethics to sustain life as long as possible. Others rather shamelessly sustain life, for which there is no hope of recovery or a return to a truly human state with little more than profit for a motive. Long-term heroic care of the dying is an extremely expensive proposition. It seems rather crass to even mention cost, but the cost we are talking about here is often so great that it could wipe out a family with a chance of many years of healthful living, a family which has definite needs for the money which is otherwise being spent in a mistaken idea of dedication to the living and sacrifice for loved ones.

Of course the question of euthanasia invariably arises when we get into this kind of discussion. There seems to be considerable pressure in its favor lately, but it is not likely that euthanasia properly so-called will find any approval officially within the Church. However, there is such a thing as "only caring" for the dying which is discussed at great length by Paul Ramsey in *The Patient as Person*.[4]

We spoke before of the new thrusts in medical ethics toward total patient care. This doesn't necessarily mean the longest possible extension of biological life. If at all possible, one who is terminally ill should be allowed a death with dignity. He should be informed of the fact that he is dying at the first moment that this is a known fact and that he is in a proper physical and mental state to receive the news. Likewise, as cold-blooded as it may seem, there appears to be a very clear-cut obligation to inform his immediate family of the true situation. Dr. Kubler-Ross insists that this helps most patients to overcome some of the terrors of death,

---

[4] Yale University Press, 1970, pp. 124-132.

among the worst uncertainty and loneliness.[5] If one knows that he is going to die, he has an opportunity to prepare himself for it spiritually and to adjust himself to it mentally. The same is true of his family and relatives. There is a growing tendency to make it possible for such patients to spend their last days at home or in other familiar surroundings. During this time, they are most certainly entitled to every possible means of making them comfortable and the most important of these may be assuring that they are never alone unless they wish to be.

Placed in the almost inevitably impersonal atmosphere of a hospital, surrounded by all kinds of machines and scurrying personnel, the man who is dying may very well suffer much more than he needs to. The old deathbed scenes of stage and screen seem quite foreign to us now for many reasons, not the least of which is disintegration of family values, but it is hard to imagine anything more Christian or more biblically oriented than the gathering of those who are closest to one as he prepares to end his sojourn on earth.

Of course it may be absolutely necessary that he be in a hospital and then the obligation arises to consider his comfort and his well-being; to support him as much as possible by understanding, not by false cheer or evasion of the fact of impending death.

Intravenous feeding would certainly not be extraordinary means under such conditions. The feeding has much the effect of a cup of cool water placed at the lips of a suffering man. Administration of pain relieving drugs, even though these could be said to hasten death, is also considered allowable by moralists.

Insofar as possible, the dying man should be given

---

[5] *Op. cit.* See also *Hospital Topics,* Spring 1972.

free choice in what he wants and what he doesn't want. Still, his mental condition, the effects of the illness on his mental processes and certain kinds of subtle coercion must be dealt with. Certainly, there is no obligation to actively prolong a life in pain when there is no hope of recovery. However, the lack of hope of recovery must be a thoroughly substantiated thing. After all, new treatments and drugs do develop and things very like "miracles" do occur. The whole thing calls for a great deal of balance in the decision making of the patient, his family and the health care team.

A great many writers in the general field see nothing at all wrong with suspending life-sustaining procedures in a case of a person who has no hope of recovery, particularly one who is comatose and not likely to recover consciousness. This would be even more so in the case of a person with sufficient brain damage to insure that recovery is impossible from any known medical point of view. There are writers who suggest that beyond termination of life prolonging procedures certain actions may be undertaken which will hasten the dying process. I believe it would be a mistake at this point to try to make any final judgment on that opinion. In any case, they are not talking about euthanasia in its usual sense. They are talking about speeding up the process of dying in one who is already in that process. Still, that leaves rather frightening judgment in human hands, and in this case extreme prudence and a great deal of consultation would seem to be minimal demands.

Mention has been made here of subtle and sometimes not so subtle coercion. A patient may be convinced that a treatment or surgical procedure is a necessary thing to preserve his life or prolong it to a beneficial degree. Such an opinion, delivered by one with the authority and status of the medical profession behind him, is, in itself, a kind of coercion and the physician certainly has an obligation to explain exactly what can be expected from the treatment and exactly what the treatment consists of. It doesn't seem very logical to encourage a patient to undergo surgery which will at best prolong a life of hopelessness and pain for a few short weeks.

In this case, all we are really talking about is the matter of extraordinary means. It has even been suggested by many that a lot of heart and transplant surgery is questionable in view of its real effects. Very few recipients of heart transplants have lived for any length of time, although there is reason to believe that the outlook may become more favorable in the future. However, patients such as those receiving the transplants are often told that this is their one last hope of continued life. If one considers that continued life may mean little more than a few weeks or months around the hospital in a hotbed atmosphere, there is a real question as to the justification of the surgery at least from the therapeutic point of view. We will consider experimentation in another chapter.

It has been suggested, too, that use of facilities and personnel and the extreme expense of certain procedures such as transplants may rob persons with every hope of recovery of the attention and care that they need. The cost of transplant surgery is staggering. The same amount of money might purchase a better quality of life for a large number of people.

Here we get into the whole matter of triage, which is best pursued in another place, but at least we can clear up one point. Our obligation is not simply to extend every last facility to the prolongation of a life which is for all practical purposes lost. The more that the patient involved meets the standard of theological death mentioned here, the more is this the case. Frequently triage decisions postpone complex, time-consuming treatment of the most seriously injured disaster victims in order to treat the greater number. There are other instances when relatively minor injuries may be treated before serious ones in order to enable persons of special qualifications or of general ability to work or do something positive in a disaster situation.

The pastoral role of the priest should be clarified a little bit by the thinking presented in this chapter. Very rarely will he be able to run to a book, look up a matter, find a few precedents and arrive at a decision that leaves him with a kind of moral certainty. Much more frequently, it will be a case of offering good human advice, based on common sense, consideration of the circumstances and a real expression of faith in clarifying the Church's teachings on death and immortality.

Obviously, the priest can be of tremendous aid to the dying person, so long as he is conscious, and his role may be even more important in dealing with the immediate family and other relatives and friends. Any priest can do a great deal to set in motion a general educational process which would help to reduce the fears and superstitions with which our society now surrounds death and dying.

The psychological factors are numberless and terribly complex, ranging from guilt to simple fear. A calm, reasoned explanation of the true situation and encouragement to follow the directions of the health care personnel, once one is assured they are thinking in the right direction, seems to be a particularly necessary pastoral task. In plain fact, it is not always attended to well in hospitals, even Catholic hospitals. A great many chaplains are content to distribute communion in the morning and annoint those in danger of death.

Visiting, consoling, instructing and praying with patients would seem to be one of the most necessary duties of the priest whether he is specifically assigned as a hospital chaplain or not. Of course, he is well advised to abide by the policies of the hospital, especially when it already has a chaplain. But motives of timidity should not keep him from bringing the best of his ministry to the people who need it most.

It's amazing what squeezing a hand or patting a shoulder will accomplish when one is visiting the sick and dying. It is amazing how much can be gained by simply listening to the family and relatives, even when this involves things which needn't be said or perhaps consists of nothing more than rambling in a difficult situation. This can be a very high form of sacrifice, simply listening to those who need to talk. Hospital personnel usually lack the time to do this and no matter how compassionate they are by nature, they may very well get in trouble by spending too much time with an individual and his family.

To sum up for the present then, there is no absolutely clear answer as to when death occurs, but there are fairly good guidelines as to when it is no longer necessary to make heroic attempts to sustain biological life. Extraordinary means which are used very frequently are rarely used because of any obligation of the patient or his family. Some physicians honestly believe they must extend every last effort to prolong life. Their views must be respected, but certainly, they should be open to discussion. We need tremendous re-education on the whole subject of death. Few people are able to view it with a truly Christian perspective. The ordinary priest is probably in the best position to tackle this job. Even as he does, he is going to have to keep abreast at least generally of medical developments and changing climates of medical opinion.

It is very true that there is a lot of genuine compassion among persons in the health care professions. There is also a lot of cynicism and a kind of hard-boiled objectivity which may have some necessary basis, but which do little to comfort the sick and the dying. Just as a phony bedside manner is no longer considered to be part of the doctor's job, everyone involved in the care and treatment of the patient, especially the dying patient, has a rather special obligation to consider his dignity, his privacy and his wishes. Again, the man who seems best suited to make these things come about is the ordinary working priest or religious.

Author's Note: Richard A. McCormick, S.J., provides an invaluable summary and evaluation of the various views of Merle Longwood, J. William Wordon, Paul Ramsey, P.R. Baelz, Arthur J. Dyck, Daniel Maguire, Joseph Fletcher, Daniel Callahan and others in "Notes on Moral Theology," *Theological Studies,* Vol. 34, No. 1 (March 1973), pp. 65-77.

5. Experimentation on Humans and Donation of Organs for Transplant

Medical research in this century has accomplished things far beyond the dreams of man. There is every reason to believe that this progress will continue and that the rate of progress will even accelerate. In practically every case of medical research some experimentation on human beings is necessary.

Under both the headings of experimentation and treatment by means of transplantation of organs we face some of the most biting questions of current medical ethics. Older writings will serve as guides to some extent, but they cannot be expected to anticipate every situation that arises. As a rule of thumb, however, it seems like a pretty good practice to review traditional decisions before undertaking a free-handed approach to any new ethical problem that may arise. Because the areas of experimentation and transplant overlap, it has been decided to treat both in one chapter, although the areas in which they do not overlap will also be treated here.

One essential principle stands out above all others and that is the sacredness of human life. This is a universal sacredness, applying to each and every human being, regardless of his state of health, his mental disposition, or his presumed worth or lack of worth to society. Paul Ramsey in *The Patient as Person* notes that there has been a casual slip from the term sacredness to the term dignity. I believe it is quite necessary to talk in terms of sacredness, although there are some areas of life and treatment in which dignity would be a better word.

The main point is that a human being, simply by virtue of his existence, has a uniqueness and a sacred character which must be respected in any and all cases. Referring to the new thrust in medical ethics toward a greater concern for total patient care, the thrust must be extended not only to the total care of some patients but to the total care of all. In practice, a great many physicians and institutions observe this kind of standard very well, but a great many others do not.

We must face the fact that as important as medical progress may be, there may be some limits beyond which experimenting is not moral and is, therefore, at least according to our teaching, not allowable. Since almost all men desire long life with as little pain as possible, we have granted a great deal of dignity and respect to the medical profession and its allied professions. This is as it should be. However, those within the medical profession are not granted any special moral character or any special judgmental ability which would separate them from the general body of professional people. Some are ethical to the point of being scrupulous, others are very casual and very cynical. A great many show no particular concern for informing the patient of the full facts in a given situation. This is sometimes justified as being consistent with good treatment because of the psychological condition of the patient and such cases certainly do exist. In general, though, if there ever was a place a man has a "right to know" it is in the realm of the treatment of the human body, especially if it happens to be his own.

So sacredness becomes a primary word in considering both experimentation and donation of organs. A second word, equally important and based on the first, is consent. While most of us would agree that there is no such thing as a perfectly free and good intention, that psychological forces and sociological conditioning have influence on any man, the purest kind of consent must be considered where experimentation on a human person is to be discussed.

In general, there are two kinds of experimentation involving human subjects. The first is the kind where the experimental procedure or treatment offers some benefit to the condition of the patient himself. The second is experimentation which has the sole purpose of adding to the body of medical knowledge. Adding to the body of medical knowledge is certainly one of our most important tasks, but it is by no means one that grants anyone absolute freedom in anything. The sacredness of the human person and the rights deriving from that far outweigh even the most pressing needs of research.

In other words, if a man has a certain disease which can be treated by established means and a physician has a wish to treat it by experimental means, a great many factors have to be considered. If the experimental means introduces new dangers, unknown variables and unpredictable side effects, it would have to offer at the same time far greater promise of cure or arrest of the condition being treated. In other words, for general purposes, the standard, ordinary procedure should be followed in ethical practice if it is an effective one. If the standard procedure offers insufficient aid in overcoming a disorder, there is every reason to consider experimental treatment. In such a case, the patient should be informed of the full situation and the balancing factors should be spelled out for him as carefully as possible. He should be fully aware of any and all risks as well as any and all unknown factors which he may face in undergoing the experimental treatment. Further, the treatment itself must offer, at least potentially, benefits in proportion to any risk, pain, discomfort or unusual expense that the patient may have to bear. If a more traditional mode of treatment offers less promise but greater safety, the patient certainly has a right to opt for it.

A rather natural desire on the part of medical personnel for progress and development and a rather natural tendency on the part of patients to seek shortcuts and miracles can often lead to unwise use of new drugs or surgical procedures. It is doubtful that very many medical men engage in what might be called unorthodox experimental practices, but they still have a rather strong motivation to advance their research wherever possible. This, coupled with the patient's desire for a quicker or more lasting remedy, could conceivably lead to some very unwise choices in relation to the sacredness of the human person. If he unwittingly submits to treatment which is more dangerous than he realizes or if the chance of improvement is less than he supposes, someone has slipped somewhere.

The point is that the patient and his family are entitled to full disclosure of facts prior to the beginning of any experimental treatment and the principle holds that the treatment must offer benefit in proportion to the risks or other negative factors involved.

As for the second kind of research and experimentation, that which is capable only of adding to the body of medical knowledge, cooperation of a patient or of any other person may be sought legitimately, but again there is a need for a highly informed kind of consent on the part of the person submitting to experimentation. To use a favorite term of Paul Ramsey's, the person may choose to become a "co-adventurer" with the medical profession in the undertaking of testing new drugs or some other kind of therapeutic procedure.[1] Again, what is called for is the fullest kind of information in advance, the greatest precautions at every stage of the procedure and moral certainty on the part of the experimenters that the subject is not being exposed to any undue risks. Certain experiments have been performed on prisoners and other voluntary personnel with some kind of due consideration involved such as monetary payment or recommendation for lessening of a sentence. In some of these cases there was at least a remote risk of death of the subjects.

I believe most moralists would hold that such research and experimentation is justifiable, so long as it conforms to the general standards of reasonable procedures, but every effort should be made to obtain a free consent from each subject who is influenced as little as possible by promise of remuneration or reduction of punishment.

Experimentation on children poses a particularly nasty situation. Many hold that it is impossible for a

[1] *The Patient as Person,* chapter 1.

sick child, or for any child for that matter, to give true consent to the undertaking of an experimental procedure upon his person. In the normal course of things, his parents would be asked for their consent just as in preparation for routine surgery. Again, a number of moralists and others considering the situation, hold that this kind of proxy consent does not have any great merit in the case of experimentation. If the experimentation is allowable at all, it would almost certainly have to be of the kind that would offer positive benefit in the treatment of some condition already existing in the child. The usual hope of profit to the person in proportion to the risk involved has to be considered and, in general, one would have to be very slow and very thoughtful in deciding that experimentation on a child is a correct and logical procedure. Very often parents who are in a distraught condition and suffering from great personal pressure and uncertainty because of a child's illness, may give a consent which they would not give if these pressures were lacking. This means that a great deal of responsibility falls upon the physician urging or requesting permission for the procedure. He certainly should be morally sure that he has a valid consent before undertaking any experimental treatment involving a child. Even then, there is some question as to the morality of the consent, it being held that the child himself almost certainly cannot give it and that his parents do not have an absolute right to give it.

This raises the question of experimentation on wards of the state. A number of rather disturbing situations have been reported where retardates or other inmates of state or other governmental institutions were used as subjects in experimentation without their knowledge. It would be very hard to justify such conduct. The child loses no rights simply because he is a ward of the state or does not have a normal family to back him up. A patient in a state hospital may have lost certain rights under civil law, but he still remains a human person, probably one who is incapable of giving consent to an experimental procedure.

What it boils down to is this, most research conducted in most places is carried out with great restraint, with careful study of possible legal liabilities and with every effort to safeguard the patient's well-being at all stages. However, our constant quest for new knowledge and our sometimes overly zealous desire to find a cure or dramatic remedy can lead to procedures which could be said to violate the sanctity of the person and the rights deriving therefrom. Such research cannot be called moral.

To bring it down to practical terms, the priest who is consulted in a case of this kind needs to do two basic things. One is to understand as thoroughly as possible just what is being proposed and how well the patient and his family understand this, and the other is to try to make the best possible judgment as to whether the research offers aid to the person or aid to the general cause of medicine in reasonable proportion to the risk the person is being asked to undertake. Again, the somewhat unhappy term "moral certainty" arises, because medicine, like all sciences, must deal in probabilities.

One of the more painful parts of our growth in the fields of ethics and moral theology is that we, too, must deal many, many times with nothing beyond moral certainty. Our absolutes are fading fast and will probably never be heard from again.

Recently, there was quite a stir over the matter of experiments on aborted fetuses. Studies of non-viable fetuses (those who cannot survive outside the womb) have been going on in England, Sweden and the United States as well as other places. The abortion products involved normally die in about an hour, but can be kept alive up to about three hours by supplying blood and air by artificial means. Many scientists state that such studies are of the utmost importance.

At this writing, the matter seems to have been pretty well checked by a decision of the National Institutes of Health not to fund any such research in the United States or abroad. The institute controls government grants to a very high percentage of existing research facilities.

There is, however, nothing to prevent such research by those who might decide to operate without government aid. Further, the really upsetting aspects of the situation lie not so much in what has already happened as in what could happen.

When an abortion is performed, the aborted fetus *(abortus)* is usually treated as a specimen or a discarded organ to be tossed in a waste bucket or placed in a jar. The mother is rarely consulted about her wishes for disposition and the Supreme Court has already ruled that a fetus less than six months old has no rights.

There is no reason to suppose that in time *aborti* couldn't be kept alive for greater lengths of time regardless of their stage of development at the time of abortion. Also, pregnancies are being terminated in the fifth and sixth months during which the *abortus* could well be able to survive alone or with a little artificial support and even brought to full term.

This raises the possibility of what is clearly human

life being used for all kinds of experimentation with little or no control. Laws are being demanded in various places, but the future of such laws is questionable. The worst of it is that we are dealing with explosive and emotional issues and just about any statement from Catholic sources is virtually guaranteed to be brushed off as reactionary in view of our general position on abortion and longstanding efforts to obtain and preserve anti-abortion laws.

It seems that the most important thing the Church could do right now is to start vigorous programs of education and action on respect for life, not just as adjuncts to campaigns to make or keep abortion illegal, but as sincere means of communicating values that would prevent at least some abortions in the first place and would make researchers more sensitive to the reality of there being some things even more important than the best research.

In cases of donation of organs by live persons for the benefit of sick persons, the same general criteria apply as to experimentation. The donor must be fully aware of what is involved, of what risks he takes and of what the potential benefit to the sick person is. Few moralists would stand in absolute opposition to the donation of organs, but almost all would be terribly careful in making sure that the proposed donation does not take the form of a useless or only slightly valuable mutilation of a human being. Probably the most common case in this area is the donation of kidneys.

Certainly as much as possible must be known about the physical and mental condition of the donor and the exact state of the potential recipient. It has been said that in cases like these it is not simply a matter of seeking a proportionate cause for the donation, but that the transplant must promise even greater benefit to the recipient than would be necessary to simply balance off the suffering, inconvenience and risk undertaken by the donor. It goes without saying that every case of this kind should be reviewed in the most thorough possible manner and in no case should the final decision be that of one or two people.

Donation of useful organs from the bodies of deceased persons is an area which allows a little bit more leeway. However, even here, there should be consent, at the very least implicit, on the part of both the patient and his family. During post-mortems, which are now common-place in most hospitals, useful organs are sometimes removed and used for various purposes. Generally speaking, this procedure is regulated by standard medical ethics and by laws applying in the area where the donation occurs. However, to be strictly moral about the matter, it would seem that a person entering a hospital where he may die should know that in the event of his death one or more organs of his body may be used for research purposes without further advertence to the matter. His family should know the same thing. If there is any reluctance on the part of either the patient or his family, their feelings should be respected to the fullest.

It is common procedure now, one which is rather widely encouraged, for persons to will their bodies or certain organs of their bodies to a medical school or other medical facility upon their death. Strictly speaking, there is no moral objection to this, but the person making such a donation of his cadaver, should do so in the most absolute kind of freedom, should not do so for monetary consideration or at least not primarily for monetary consideration, and should have the right to specify any restrictions which he wishes to place on the use of the cadaver. He should also have the right to cancel his agreement for disposition of his body at any time. There are those who hold, and I think that I would agree with them, that members of the immediate family should have at least something to say about the final disposition of the body and that if there is sufficient objection, agreements for donation should be cancelled.

One reason for this is that while there are standard forms which take into consideration just about any ethical aspect one could wish, people are notoriously poor at reading small print. Caught up in the sentiment or feeling of heroism that might accompany completion of such a form and the signing away the rights to one's body after death, one may overlook a great many of the procedures which people of good intention have built into the form itself. Very often, the agreement that is actually made simply gives the cadaver to a hospital or medical school with no restrictions. I am sure there have been many cases where a person has approached death feeling that his body will be used for some good and worthwhile purpose such as the curing or at least successful treatment of a living person.

This is not always the case. There is generally a shortage of bodies for use in the laboratory study of gross anatomy, and a cadaver may simply be turned over to students for dissection, a prospect which the donor may never have contemplated fully and might well have rejected if he had.

It could certainly be said that there is a definite benefit to mankind in having cadavers for medical students to study, but placed on any normal scale of values it would seem that this value is less than the value of donation of an organ for the treatment of a living person.

Again it comes down to clear knowledge of what is proposed and intended and clear, unobstructed and uncoerced consent on the part of the donor.

The whole business of willing away one's body strikes me a little wrong for some reason, even though I can see all kinds of values to be derived. But sometimes the theorist has to leave his office or study or lab and look at things as they actually are. Having spent some time around cadaver rooms, having watched the handling of cadavers in medical schools, and having been present at any number of post-mortems and medical school dissections, I have a little quirk. That is that I do not wish my remains to be used in this manner, no matter how important the results might be. I would look at the donation of one of my eyes or of some other organ in a much different way. This is purely personal.

The final point is that there is no strict moral objection to the donation of organs either by the living or the dead. But in all such cases a great deal of thought must be given to precisely what is being undertaken, to what the potential benefits are and what the potential disvalues may be. Further, the clearest possible consent from anyone involved should be obtained. This is only a personal opinion, but I think that in the case of organ donation, the families of donors have certain rights, albeit less than final. I believe they should be consulted, fully informed and that their views should at least be given a good hearing before any final decision is made.

I know from personal experience that autopsy consents are frequently obtained in ways which are legal but less than lofty and some of my own relatives have on occasion obtained specimens from cadavers which the cadaver before death would not agree to and which the family strongly opposed. There is a general feeling among researchers that we must do everything we can do and advance as far and as fast as we can. For a great many people in the sciences, this constitutes their working morality. To say the least, it is less than complete. The sanctity of human life and of the human person, even a dead person, demands just a little bit more consideration, reflection and delicacy in action. I do not believe that this is the kind of thinking that will hamper research greatly, in fact it may add to its dignity. In any case I will not allow it to be attacked as being a sentimental reaction. Several authors note that the horrible procedures undertaken in medical research during the Nazi reign began with the use of persons considered to be beyond rehabilitation, then considered to be "useless" persons.

I don't believe that we can follow a domino theory in all things and say that failure to use extraordinary means to preserve the life of a hopelessly sick person is automatically an open door to euthanasia. Nor do I think that relaxing our views on contraception or sterilization or even abortion in highly selected cases is opening the door to all kinds of abuse or immorality.

On the other hand, I am aware of the potential for cynicism among persons who are closely connected with the care of the sick and the dying and those who are involved in research and experimentation. It isn't even a culpable cynicism. In most cases it is a kind of hardening that comes with time and experience.

That does not mean that we shouldn't stop every once in awhile and do a little thinking and reflecting to make sure that things aren't getting out of hand. Most of the monstrous activities of man in the research field had their beginnings in relatively small, seemingly unobjectionable ways. The domino theory is neither a universal nor an absolute, but it is always worth considering.

Author's Note: A complete reading of Paul Ramsey's *The Patient as Person* on this subject is practically essential and will expose the reader to various degrees and directions of thought from diverse sources.

6. Genetic Engineering, Genetic Surgery and Artificial Insemination

It is virtually impossible to write anything definitive on the subject of genetic engineering and genetic surgery at this time because we are dealing almost entirely with possibilities, although in some cases reasonable probabilities. As these possibilities and probabilities approach frightening proportions, they raise the possibility of future ethical and moral decisions for which there is no precedent in all of history.

To put it simply, it appears that within ten or twenty years men may be able to do practically anything in terms of making or rearranging other men. There has already been considerable laboratory success with asexual reproduction and it is not at all impossible that we might actually produce a man by asexual means in the reasonably near future.

The basic procedure involves placing the nucleus from a human cell in an unfertilized ovum. It is called cloning, which means simply cutting. Embryonic life could be sustained *in vitro* (in test tubes or similar devices) and at a given time implanted in a mother or host, if you will. It is even possible that men might be made and undergo their entire embryonic and fetal existence without a human mother playing any role. Few have suggested this very seriously, but the entire field offers such a wide range of science fiction-type possibilities that one really shouldn't rule out anything.

Through various techniques of genetic engineering and genetic surgery, it should be possible to make people to order, to determine the length of their arms or their legs or the degree of their intelligence. It has even been suggested in one novel that the male sex might be eliminated altogether and a kind of female utopia created.

It must be noted that all of this is in the realm of speculation and that no one can seriously blame any researchers who have simply sought to know as much as possible about the genetic composition of man and the possibilities of managing it. The question that arises is: To what extent should man manage man?

What are the rights of the population in general? What are the rights of any human person to have it determined by another human person that he cannot reproduce or that he should reproduce in a given way? These are only a few of the very haunting questions that arise.

Many moralists I know are inclined to postpone serious thinking on the matter beyond occasional speculation on the grounds that all we really have are possibilities and a lot of very interesting research. It should be noted, however, that those involved in research sometimes express a kind of grandiose philosophy in which they come very close to playing God. It is a legitimate thing to be concerned with the genetic pool—and the way that it might be used to best advantage. However, one moves very quickly from this to deciding what kind of people should be and what kind of people shouldn't be. It is entirely possible for a scientist of the not too distant future to be in a position to make such a decision.

Because man is, among other things, a political animal and a product that we refer to as "the fall of man," it is very easy to become disturbed about the possibilitiy that the nature and quality of life might be placed entirely in human hands.

One might very well argue that that's the way it is now except we don't manage it very well. It would be hard to argue with the observation that if breeders allowed livestock to breed as carelessly and in some cases as foolishly as men do we would have very inadequate and very poor livestock indeed. But we are not talking about livestock, we are talking about human beings and the question arises: To what extent does a man have a right to determine what the nature or composition of another man will be?

We are confronted at many stages in the consideration of genetic planning with a kind of scientific utopian point of view. There are those who argue that their concern is not the gene pool at all but the total good of mankind. It isn't terribly hard to grant that most people who talk in these terms talk from very lofty motives. The question remains, and it haunts religious thinkers: To what extent is man limited or should man be limited in such undertakings? Is life a kind of colossal joke, a kind of genetic crap game or is it in some way a plan of God? Certainly there is nothing wrong with trying to improve the quality of human beings and the quality of their life. That is the basis of almost all research. But when it comes down to the reproduction of human beings who are presumed by Christians to have immortal souls, albeit a rather different kind of souls than we thought about in former hellenistic terms, the matter becomes a great deal stickier.

A statement frequently heard in connection with this is: "Man should do what man can do." It sounds good and in some cases it seems to have a kind of inescapable logic. The fact is that man can blow up the world; it can hardly be argued that he should therefore do so.

Of course, geneticists and other researchers concerned with the quality of reproduction are not talking about blowing up the world but improving the world. Unfortunately that's pretty much what they had in mind when they started atomic research. The awful threat of nuclear annihilation that hovers over man today did not spring from minds that were bent on the destruction of man and his world. Very few research scientists are evil men. All we are left with is a terrible question for which there is no immediate answer: To what extent can man morally control mankind?

On a less exotic and less speculative level it can certainly be said that genetic screening of humans contemplating marriage could be a very good thing. Whether or not a human person has an ethical obligation to submit to such screening is, at this point at least, an open question. It would seem that a man with the best interests of man at heart would want to know what the possibilities of his marrying a given woman might be, what good or what harm might result from their reproducing. As noted previously, it seems like a very good idea to know before marriage what these possibilities are and, if they are serious enough, to make some kind of plans to avoid damaging mankind by producing defectives.

The somewhat sentimental argument that even defectives may have a place in God's scheme of things is not quite as foolish as it sounds. I find it hard to buy personally, but I do believe that God made the world and I do believe that God made mankind as it is. I have very great reservations as to how much I think man should tamper with this. At the same time I believe that we have a moral obligation to pursue research in all areas as diligently as possible. The result comes very close to being a perfect dilemma.

This much is so. Thinkers in all fields, not just theology, but law, medicine, economics, every scholarly dicipline now existing, have an obligation to anticipate the kinds of questions that are virtually certain to arise from current genetic experimentation. We really should have an answer as to whether or not a person should be required to have genetic screening prior to marriage as he is required to now have a Wasserman test in most places.

Assuming that the genetic screening produces a negative picture, we are confronted with some very searching questions in terms of man's freedom and in terms of man imposing what he takes to be the common good as a ground for forbidding reproduction in certain cases. Once a defective has resulted from a marriage, a certain amount of counseling seems to be in order. This is going to raise a great many questions regarding contraception, sterilization and, perhaps, abortion. All we can do now is look at the possibilities.

At the same time, we have to realize that the human population is subject to more control by man than ever before and that this control will grow. It is in itself a product of human intelligence and human intelligence was made by God. I would hate to be guilty of offering a very simple answer to the immense complex of questions that arises.

The ordinary priest to whom this book is addressed will probably have to limit himself to this same kind of running in circles. In fact, the questions don't have to be answered now, and really there are no answers now since we do not yet have full questions. About the only thing that is certain is that just as research is proceeding at a very rapid clip, ethical and moral speculation must make every effort to stay abreast of the field and try to arrive at some reasonable consensus. The man in the laboratory has his own brand of morality. Frequently it is highly motivated. Whether that is enough to allow any man to proceed with the notion that man should do what man can do is quite another matter.

The area of artificial insemination is a little bit easier to deal with. The traditional Catholic position remains pretty much intact. The medical profession has learned to do a great deal to increase fertility of couples who are having difficulty having children. The Church has been rather insistent that this be carried out to the greatest possible extent according to the "normal" or "natural" means of sexual reproduction. That is to say, a physician may aid a couple so that the chances of having a child are at a maximum. There remains a great deal of reservation in the whole area. A certain amount of liberalization seems inevitable.

What seems just about equally certain is that artificial insemination by donated semen other than that of a woman's husband will remain as it is now considered immoral in formal church teaching. There is very little likelihood of any official change in position, and there are some pretty good scientific reasons for avoiding what is known as A.I.D. (Artificial insemination, donor). The problem is that if two women are fertilized by semen from the same donor, and this is a distinct possibility when semen is drawn from a bank, there remains a possibility of their offspring unknowingly becoming involved in marriage and reproducing what may prove to be very defective offspring. It is a kind of inbreeding of the worst kind. It has been suggested that women who have been fertilized in this manner somehow mark themselves or their children so that the possibility of their offspring falling in love and re-producing would be kept to an absolute minimum. There doesn't really seem to be any practical way of doing this at the present time. What seems to be quite certain is that from a standpoint of Christian ethics, the use of donated semen for purposes of artificial insemination may present very grave dangers in addition to the moral objections that were there in the first place.

There is no question that there is rapidly growing approval of artificial insemination and this includes approval by Catholic physicians and theologians. I know quite a few physicians who would not hesitate to use artificial insemination of donated semen in any case that they thought would be aided substantially by this process.

The theological opinion relating to the matter is admittedly one held by a minority. It holds that if we seek a total morality, that is the total good of all persons involved as well as the good of society, there is no substantial moral objection in selected cases to artificial insemination using donated semen.

In the cases where this is approved by Catholic theologians, a major medical center is usually involved, an example being the University of Michigan. Here, after studying all aspects of the case, staff members will pursue the idea of artificial insemination by donor likelihood of any official change in position, and there but insist on a long period of intensive counseling of husband and wife. If all concerned are satisfied that the procedure will work to the total advantage of both parties so far as can be foreseen and if the psychological counseling results are satisfactory, donated semen is then used and the woman is artificially inseminated.

Commenting on the objection that there may be severe genetic dangers in the use of donated semen from banks, one physician expressed the opinion that the odds involved are really not much worse than the day-to-day possibilities and percentages in the general population.

For purposes of pastoral counseling, there is little need for discussion. A woman can go to a legitimate fertility clinic in good conscience. She and her husband may be treated in various ways so that they have a maximum chance of producing good healthy offspring. Near miracles have been worked in this field and there is a great deal of reason to hope for even more important developments in the future. However, a woman must certainly be warned against the possible dangers of artificial insemination by means of semen from a bank. Some leading thinkers in the field have proposed that an absolute moratorium on the whole business be declared because of the dangers that arise not only ethically but biologically.

It would have been nice to have presented a perfectly clear step-by-step chapter on these subjects. It must be obvious that there is no clear guide to give. In the whole area of genetic engineering, genetic surgery and artificial insemination, the priest may feel bound to a rather static position. About all he can do is keep informed of new developments and see which of these, if any, fall within the normal range of ethical or moral activity. Genetic research can be called a moral good, but the use of the findings of genetic research could very possibly lead to a moral catastrophe. Medical efforts to improve fertility are certainly a moral good, assuming that they are carried on in a reasonable and ethical fashion. Because of the possibilities of real damage resulting from uncontrolled use of semen banks, it is a very safe thing to simply caution against this kind of insemination no matter how badly one wants a child. Many will disagree with that statement.

From a pastoral point of view one is left with two choices. One is to refer a couple who wishes a child but has had difficulty in having one to the most reputable and ethical fertility clinic he knows. The other is to consider the possibility of adoption. It is no news to anyone that there are a great many unwanted children who would like homes very much. Although it doesn't seem quite the same to take someone else's child and raise it as one's own, most people who have done this have found it a rewarding experience which in many ways equals the full experience of parenthood.

The only remaining admonition that one can offer is that it is going to be necessary for anyone concerned with ethics and morals to stay abreast of all developments in the fields of genetic engineering and surgery, of fertility therapy, of anything having to do with new or improved or different means of reproduction. This is not easy to do. Fortunately, the popular and semischolarly press have caught up with the issue and there is every reason to believe that there will be a fair amount of information available to the diligent reader.

There remains the terrible challenge to scholars in the fields of ethics and morality to do more than keep abreast of actual developments. Theirs is the frightening job of anticipating what questions may arise and trying to work out answers to them.

Author's Note: For discussion of various issues in this chapter, see also *Fabricated Man,* Paul Ramsey, Yale University Press and *Theological Studies,* Vol. 33, No. 3 (Fall 1972). Further valuable reflection will be found in the article, "Technology Assessment and Genetic Engineering," by John J. Carey in *Theological Studies,* Vol. 33, No. 4 (Dec. 1972).

7. The Changing Physician-Patient Relationship

If you would like a medical ethic that would please the great majority of the members of the profession, it would be based on the premise that the professional decision of a fully qualified physician in a given matter *is* the ethical decision.

It may sound like a simplistic approach, but actually there is something to recommend it. A physician has had to earn his degree the hard way and in order to become licensed he has had to pass through an internship and pass licensure examinations. A large number of physicians now practicing have resident training beyond that, backed up by continued study and occasional return to formal post-graduate study.

They have had to earn their right to privileges on the staffs of the hospitals in which they practice and they practice under continual supervision of various hospital and professional committees. They must constantly consider the legal ramifications of every action they undertake. By all normal standards, the ordinary practicing physician could be said to be an ethical professional man operating within a framework which guarantees to a large extent that his practice will be an ethical one.

However, there are still many ways in which the most ethical physician or surgeon can err in his judgments and there will always be a few unscrupulous or less than fully moral members of the profession. It is never a very good idea to leave highly complicated ethical decisions in the hands of one man or even a small group of colleagues. The matter is further complicated (and this is the dominant argument against the kind of ethical freedom many doctors would like) because the relationship between the doctor and his patient has been changing and is virtually certain to change a great deal more.

No amount of lamenting will restore the old "family doctor." Most people who can afford it have a general practitioner or an internist who fills to some extent the family doctor role. A few years ago it was suggested that such practitioners be regarded as "family health care managers." That is to say, they would handle routine problems, build up the best possible medical knowledge of all members of the family and make the proper referrals to specialists when these were needed. This is a fairly practical approach even at the present time, but it is not wholly adequate and there are conditions to suggest that something much more than a man designated as health care manager will be needed in the future.

The reason for this goes beyond the continuing trend toward specialization within the medical field. More and more men are turning to specialties and more and more specialties are turning up. There is a certain crossover here, in that men in various specialties do practice to some extent outside those specialties.

The big point is the series of changes which economic factors are causing in the profession. The economics involved come from both the doctor's side and the patient's side.

Group practice is for many physicians and surgeons the only possible way to provide adequate service to the residents of their communities. A few internists and general practioners working in collaboration with a surgeon or two, an OB-GYN man, perhaps a gastroenterologist, an EENT man and even a psychiatrist can afford to have a medical center which can allow much of their practice to be conducted within one building. They can afford their own X-ray equipment, labs and other diagnostic devices and the personnel to man them. The business management of the group practice is a great deal more practical than the office management of a single physician. Generally both the doctor and the patient find the arrangement better than the single practitioner office which still is probably the most common setup in the United States. It is possible for the members of the group to cover each other to allow for a certain amount of time off and to make sure someone is available to take care of night and weekend calls. The non-surgeons in the group frequently assist the surgeons, thereby solving a problem of having competent assistance in communities where interns and residents are not available.

Still, while the person who deals with a practicing group usually claims one member of the group as his own doctor, he has a less intensive relationship with this doctor than he would have had with the old-time family physician. The efficiency that is gained through group practice very often is reduced to a time and motion study and the patient rarely has time for a leisurely consultation with a doctor, often does not have time to ask the very question he came in to have answered. He also finds himself dealing from time to time with a doctor he doesn't know.

The same general conditions prevail in prepaid medical plans where the emphasis is on preventive medicine and continuation of good health as well as on treating individual ailments as they arise. A patient may be assigned to one or another doctor and may even have some choice in the matter, but, in fact, he rarely has a direct, fixed relationship with an individual physician.

Recently, Dr. Andre Hellegers stated very strongly that having seen the advent of socialized medicine in the Netherlands and in England, he was completely convinced that some form of government medicine was inevitable in this country and that its arrival was not too far off.[1] Yet, even under such programs, the patient often has some choice of doctors. Still, under any of the circumstances described here, it is no longer a one-to-one relationship and there is every indication that it will become less and less a one-to-one relationship as time goes on.

Of course, the ever-increasing role of government in both health care and research presents many troubling questions. Government involvement in research, including research with human subjects, causes grave concern when you consider that as much as eighty percent of the funding for biomedical studies comes from government sources.

There are those who fear that this could lead to

---

[1] During a Conference on the Ethical and Religious Directives for Health Care Facilities, held at Mercy Center, Farmington, Michigan, April 1972.

the government's having the market cornered on extremely sensitive scientific knowledge which could be misused in any number of ways. The ethical questions here border on the infinite.

Another fear arises from the fact that government medical training grants are due to be terminated in 1974. These have been viewed as a quality control factor since there was great care taken to make sure that training conducted under these included careful exposure of benefactors to ethical considerations. There are reliable observers who say that sponsored research will continue, but may fall into the hands of persons not thus schooled.

The principal worry, however, is in the direct area of everyday medical practice which we are discussing here. Any great increase in a "Big Brother" atmosphere in the health care field could lead to changes, restraints, cautions and restrictions conceivable only to those who really know bureaucracy first-hand. Patient privacy, which we will consider in a later chapter, is only one area of concern.

Up-tight practitioners is another. Even now, with malpractice suits being what they are, I know of physicians who will not tell patients they are pregnant until there are certain signs, such as fetal heart beat. They simply report that tests were positive and the uterus shows such and such enlargement. Imagine what would happen if a practitioner knew full well that federal inspectors of one kind or another had full access to knowledge of every phase of his professional activities.[2]

What does this mean in terms of ethics and morality? The patient who had one doctor who took care of

[2] See Stephen Strickland, *Politics, Science and Dread Disease* (Harvard University Press).

most of his medical needs was well known to the doctor and had a pretty good knowledge of the doctor himself. The doctor had a reasonable notion of what the patient's outlook was, what his religious convictions were and what his wishes for his family and himself might be under most conditions. The patient, on the other hand, was sufficiently acquainted with the doctor to know what his convictions were and the direction of care he was apt to provide. Above all, he felt free to discuss preferences, likes and dislikes with such a doctor, could count on him for the most part for full information in any given set of circumstances and could be reasonably sure any treatment given himself or any member of his family was treatment that was freely chosen.

For instance, the ordinary Catholic, with his own doctor, regardless of the doctor's religion, could be quite sure that the doctor would respect his wishes in regard to any moral issues that might arise in the course of his care. The doctor, in short, was not apt to suggest an abortion even when one might be legal or to recommend sterilization or a number of other procedures clearly known to be in conflict with the wishes of most Catholics.

He might mention these as alternatives, but would almost always be sure to inform the patient well in advance of any contemplated actions that might result in a moral conflict and even to help him in resolving the conflict. The ordinary Catholic going to the ordinary Catholic doctor had quite reasonable certainties as to the course the doctor would follow in ethical and moral matters.

Even in the case of a patient-physician relationship where there was no definite religious affiliation on either side, there was a sufficient personal relationship to assure that the convictions of the patient and the convictions of the physician would not collide head-on, that there would be respect for both and that any real conflicts would be resolved.

In an emergency situation, a physician who knows a patient well can be counted on to avoid procedures which he knows would be abhorrent to the patient and to follow procedures which he knows the patient would generally favor.

As the individual patient becomes the concern of more and more doctors, this kind of relationship decreases very rapidly. Within the members of a group practice, certain general policies and practices do prevail, but a patient can never be sure that the member of the group caring for him as a substitute for another member of the group knows and will respect his choices in given matters as would the doctor he deals with primarily. The bigger the group or the bigger the health care center in which the patient finds himself, the more this is the case.

Generally a physician will refer a patient to a surgeon who will be reasonably well informed of the patient's moral preferences and generally the surgeon can be counted on to respect these. But the more distant the relationship becomes between the patient and the practitioner or even between the referring physician or other specialists, the less this is so. To be sure, there are broad areas of medical ethics in which there will be little difference in the approach of one man from another. But there are all kinds of choices which can and must be made, sometimes in a great hurry. The less intimately connected the doctor and patient are, the greater the odds seem to be that the physician may select a course which is not the one the patient would choose if he had full information and full opportunity to make a choice.

Choice becomes a terribly important word in the practice of medicine these days. In day-to-day practice, most of the choices are made by the doctors and the patients are then informed. Only when the patient's full consent is required to follow a procedure legally, is the patient consulted to any great degree. The amount of consultation that takes place depends a great deal on the individual doctor and many do not feel any particular obligation to spend the amount of time necessary to insure this. In fact, time is the enemy in almost every case.

A great deal of treatment in all branches of medicine is carried out very quickly with very little reflection on anybody's part. The doctor makes his diagnosis, decides on a course of treatment and orders it. Often the patient has no idea at all of what is going on. For the most part, this does not pose any serious problems except that the patient does have a very fundamental right to know what is happening to him and why.

Generally speaking, only the doctor has the full authority to tell him. Nurses and others attending him are restricted as to the amount of information they can give and for all practical purposes are forbidden to give anything but general advice to go along with the prescribed treatment.

In other words, a patient who is suddenly stricken may find himself under the care of one or more doctors whom he does not know at all. He has no way of evaluating their competence, no way of knowing what their general philosophy of practice is. The more that the matter falls under the heading of emergency, the less he or any one of his family is apt to be consulted unless such consultation is absolutely required in order for the doctor or doctors to stay within the law or the policies of a hospital. In most cases a patient signs a consent form upon admission to a hospital which authorizes practically any treatment, including surgery, that may be required by the doctor in charge of the case. From that point on, the patient has little or no free will. He may resist and complain, but usually it will do him little or no good. Rarely does he understand his own rights as to refusal of certain treatments and procedures. Here are a few examples.

A woman in a New York City apartment building had been suffering from severe headaches for a couple of days. She did not have a regular physician so she went to the office of a "physician and surgeon" in the building. He examined her, told her she had the next thing to acute appendicitis and should go to the hospital at once. She was startled and confused by this advice, but afraid not to follow it, and within a few hours found herself in a hospital bed and prepared for "emergency" surgery.

It was a busy day in the hospital and she was not seen by a member of the house staff until shortly before she was due to go to the operating room. Fortunately, a surgical resident visited her before she was heavily sedated and she explained the situation to him. After examining her, he told her that in his own opinion she did not have appendicitis and there was nothing in the laboratory findings to indicate that she did. He advised her of her right to "sign herself out." A half hour later, the woman was back in street clothes, and back on the street. She still had the headache, but she also still had her appendix and undoubtedly saved herself several hundred dollars.

Within the profession, the exact handling of the matter by the resident could be a matter for some discussion, since he took it upon himself to contradict her "attending physician." However, the "physician and surgeon" did not choose to press the matter.

It frequently happens that after a severe emotional crisis a patient will enter a public or private "mental institution" or the psychiatric section of a general hospital of his own free will or upon the advice of a physician. Quite often, such a patient soon decides that he is not as bad off as he thought and does not wish to pursue furthur psychiatric treatment. He may be right or wrong, but he may also find himself in a situation he never dreamed of. By admitting himself he may have given the institution the legal right to hold him for a brief period of time, ranging from 24 hours to several days depending on the laws of the state. Many will insist on the patient's remaining for this minimum period. The point is, the patient, whatever his condition, should have been informed of this situation in advance or, if he could not have understood it at the time, it should have been made perfectly clear to his family. Very often this is not done.

While there is rarely bad will or immoral intent involved, it is almost a rule of thumb that the more distant the relationship between the doctor and the patient, the less freedom of choice the patient has. It is a basically fundamental teaching that the patient should have the fullest possible choice at all times. There are all kinds of court cases which lead in all kinds of directions, but the basic principle remains that, allowing for a few possible exceptions, the patient has every right to accept or decline treatment as offered. Very few patients know this.

A great many people assume that once they enter a doctor's office or a hospital they have to do as they are told. Most of the time, going along with this will do little harm to anyone and is probably the best course to take. However, this is by no means a universal.

Not too long ago, moralists would excuse from obligations to treatment a "maiden" who experienced repugnance at the possibility of treatment by a male physician. One rarely thinks of repugnance of maidens anymore, and most maidens will promptly strip on command. The point is they don't have to. Similarly, the privacy of a male patient is something that must be considered. It is often a matter of little concern to medical and hospital personnel in general, hardened as they are to the realities of everyday diagnosis and treatment, and respectful as they usually are of human persons.

In fact, in many cases the fault lies more with the patient who is lacking a sufficient sense of his own rights and privacy and a sufficient knowledge of how to enforce them than it does with the medical personnel who can usually be presumed to be functioning in good faith. But there are ethical and moral questions. The sacredness of the human person does prevail. It is threatened more and more by an increasingly casual relationship between doctor and patient or, better yet, the patient and the various doctors he will encounter in the course of his treatment.

From a pastoral point of view, it appears that there would be few serious and urgent problems here, but, in general, it seems like a good idea to make sure that anyone under one's care has at least a basic knowledge of his moral rights, legal options and fundamental choices as he goes about caring for his health and overseeing the care of the members of his family. Few priests like the image of the old time cleric or nun peering down over his shoulder as the doctor goes about his work. By the same token, there would seem to be a pastoral obligation to educate and reeducate medical personnel with which one comes into contact on the whole matter of the sacredness of the human person, of his rights to choice and of the general line of medical care that those he serves as pastor or associate pastor desire.

It will do him litle good to pontificate, but it might help him a little to philosophize occasionally with members of the medical profession. When they have the time and opportunity, and they do no matter what they tell you, they often welcome such conversation. Many are terribly aware of the speed at which they must work to get everything done and many have fairly serious questions as to the ways to handle various situations. Few will welcome imposed decisions. Many will welcome understanding dialogue.

Lack of time for thoughtful discussions with patients or clients is by no means limited to the medical profession. Many attorneys deal much too swiftly with their clients and the same could be said of accountants and others who presume that their expertise is the thing sought by their client, not their understanding of his personal wishes. With few exceptions, this is not the way most doctors really want it. The priest might be quite surprised to find that they are more than willing to listen to him and their listening may do a great deal to solve the mounting problems of the changing doctor-patient relationship.

8. Decisions, Decisions
and Tougher Decisions

At the same time that he called for better understanding of the changing patient-physician relationship, Dr. Hellegers said it was necessary to distinguish between decisions made under emergency conditions and those made when there is ample time for consultation and reflection.[1]

Commenting on this, Sister Mary Janice Belen asked: "What is an emergency?"[2]

For our present purposes, let us define two kinds of emergencies. The first is one involving an individual patient or a small number of patients following an accident or the sudden acute onset of serious symptoms. It is usually faced either in a hospital emergency room or in the field. In this kind of case we can refer to an emergency as a situation in which failure to take quick action in inaugurating certain procedures would certainly result in the death of a patient or of his progressing to a condition which would be seriously and more or less permanently damaging. Almost always, given

---

[1] During a Conference on the Ethical and Religious Directives for Health Care Facilities, held at Mercy Center, Farmington, Michigan, April 1972.

[2] In a personal communication to the author.

these conditions, there is very little opportunity to confer with the patient and not much opportunity for physicians to confer with one another. That being so, this is probably a case where the decision of a competent, established physician has to be viewed as the ethical one, assuming that he functions within the normal borders of medical practice.

A second kind of emergency is that which involves a large number of persons, such as a flood, tornado or other major disaster. In such cases the word "triage" comes into play. The standard procedure is for one doctor to be designated as triage officer. He makes all decisions as to who will be treated and how; his decisions are followed more or less automatically. Generally, there is no time for argument or discussion.

Triage decisions are dangerous and filled with possibilities for error and the triage officer occupies an unenviable position. In general, he will set aside the most serious cases, determine as best he can the common good, and what best serves that, and order treatment accordingly. In other words, if the disaster conditions are still in progress, as in the case of a flood, he may postpone treatment of the most seriously ill in order to treat a great number of persons who may be of service in controlling disaster conditions or in aiding in the treatment of others. In such cases, authors prefer a broader notion of the common good, and leave little room for the measurement of the particular worth of the persons being treated, allowing for the fact that there are special instances such as treating a physician first in order that he may treat others. Aside from cases like that, absolute equality must be presumed and the social worth and status of the person being treated are not legitimate considerations.

Even when there is no great question of returning men to active service in combating disaster conditions or aiding in the treatment of patients, cases requiring the most facilities and the greatest use of available personnel may be set aside so that the greatest number may be treated. This is a delicate kind of decision, one which leaves the triage officer a very lonely man. He may also find himself in the position of deciding that certain cases are beyond help and set these aside in order to treat the most serious victims with a reasonable chance for recovery. In general, most authors are insistent upon an absolute equality of patients.

The only time when this equality may be prescinded from is the kind of case in which the whole situation may be reduced to a limited, clearly defined objective which involves all of those concerned. Such a case is in the United States Army records dating back to 1943 during a heavy battle. There was a great shortage of penicillin and a great need for it. There were many battle casualties and many victims of venereal disease. The decision was made to use the penicillin for the treatment of the "brothel wounded" because they could be cured more quickly and restored to active duty on the battle lines. A review of the case upheld the decision. [3]

The distribution of sparse supplies and personnel and the questions involved extend all the way to who shall live and who shall die. Again, the presumption is that all men are exactly equal and that no factor other than their need for help is to be considered unless restoring them to health or ability to function serves some specific and urgent common goal.

There comes the question as to how supplies and

---

[3] Reported by Paul Ramsey, *The Patient as Person*, p. 257.

personnel should be used when it is certain that some will suffer because they are denied either the supplies or the personnel to give treatment. The decisions here become harder and harder as the severity of the situation increases.

Perhaps it's just as well to jump ahead to the ultimate question of life and death, draw what conclusions we can come to from these and then give some thought to less dramatic situations.

At the present time it is quite common to decide who will or will not be allowed the use of kidney machines for dialysis until such time as they can receive a kidney transplant. In most cases, denial of the use of a machine amounts to the decision that the patient will die. A wide number of suggestions exist as to how to face the questions involved and sometimes it has come down to employing a "life and death" committee.

It is generally presumed that members of such a committee should not be members of the medical profession. The doctor's role is to recommend a patient for the machine and explain why he believes the treatment will be beneficial in a particular case and why he believes it should be extended to a particular patient. From that point on, a doctor's judgment is in no way superior to the judgment of any other reasonably intelligent and concerned group, although the group is usually able to call upon doctors who are "neutral parties" for specific technical advice.

In a typical instance, eighteen or twenty cases might be presented by various doctors to a committee when facilities for treatment are available for only ten. This means for all practical purposes that about half of the patients involved will be left to die by the decisions of the committee.

In the case of dialysis, a certain amount of pre-screening is done. In a typical case children are often ruled out on the grounds that they are unable to tolerate long treatment on the machine and will not mature properly while receiving the treatment. Persons over forty-five are generally ruled out because of limited chances of success. Likewise, those whose conditions are complicated by other diseases or who seem to be psychologically or temperamentally unable to endure the treatment are screened out. Presumably, then, the committee receives proposed patients who will receive maximum benefit from the use of the machine and has to choose which of these will actually get the treatment. One defect in the prescreening system is that it is only natural that some doctors present their cases and assemble references better than others and this may affect the committee's decision.

The committee is presented with as much data as possible, except for the actual identity of the patient. Then the job of selecting begins. Here, as in triage decisions, the principle of the greatest good for the greatest number of people is often the guiding factor although this by no means is universally embraced by ethicists. Judgments are based on many considerations such as number of dependents, importance of the individual to the community, the projected contributions of the patient to the community, etc.

Many authors addressing themselves to the subject find the whole procedure abhorrent. Basically, what it comes down to is selecting those who will live on the basis of their supposed social worth. This recalls an old Mort Sahl monologue about airline drama. It was necessary for several persons to jump from the plane in order to keep it in flight, and the decision was made to have passengers jump in inverse relationship to their social worth. Sahl commented: "There was this terrific argument between a disc jockey and a used car salesman."

The point is that social worth is a hard thing to determine and that a patient's social worth today may mean little tomorrow. Suppose a man were chosen because he lived a good religious life. This would mean little if he ceased to live a good religious life upon commencement of treatment. Suppose a man were selected because of his potential contributions to the arts. There is nothing to guarantee that he will make such contributions. You will note that I have instinctively referred to men. There are figures that would seem to indicate that men will come out better than women when their cases are presented to such committees. In part, this is due to the fact that doctors seem to present more male cases than female cases in the first place.

In any case, all of the intangibles, all of the imponderables, are omitted, leaving a great deal of room for the prejudices, assumptions and preconditioning of the members of the committee. However neutral they may appear, such factors affect their decisions as to who shall die. All in all, the committee approach, as hallowed as it is in our society, does not appeal to many ethical and moral thinkers.

What then do we do? Ramsey[4] and others have explored civil and maritime law and a great many situations, some very complicated and well outside the medical field, in a quest for guiding principles. The two which seem to be most prominent, although by no means most favored, are taking patients for procedures

[4] *Ibid.,* p. 260.

such as dialysis on a first-come-first-served basis or else deciding who shall live and who shall die by some random selection such as casting lots.

There is a school of thought which says simply: "When all cannot be saved, all must perish." Whatever the merits of that approach, it doesn't offer much of a solution to us. Few would be inclined to abandon treatment such as dialysis simply because it is not available to all.

Ramsey[5] and others reflect upon a religiously based notion that the real decision in many cases could be made by a person who is willing to give up his chances at the machine or the use of some other sparse materials and personnel so that someone else may live. They point out that most Americans have an absolute terror of death and believe that technological sustaining of life is almost a basic right. A person of truly deep ideals who believes that death is not the worst thing a man can face, may eliminate many of the life-and-death questions or at least reduce their number by voluntarily foregoing the treatment. It is not inconceivable that such an option might be presented by the priest to the person he is counseling, although he could by no means urge it as the only possible moral choice.

Then there's a suggestion by a great many authors that reordering of our priorities is essential and that it is much more important to use the funds and personnel employed in extreme procedures such as dialysis for the treatment of a greater number of persons who have little or no hope of treatment for more ordinary conditions. It is suggested that this reordering of priorities could even move outside the medical field and consider the employment of funds and resources for urban

---

[5] *Ibid.*, chapter 7.

development, relief of poverty and many other social goals.

The consensus seems to be that procedures such as dialysis and transplants will probably have to coexist with the reordering of priorities and that means that the life and death decisions will remain.

If anything can be said to be ethically and morally objectionable in the whole matter it would be in the committee-style selection of patients for treatment based on social value. Beyond that, there are many possible options. Members of the medical profession and administrators of health care facilities can go in any of a number of directions without encountering a just charge of negligence or inhumanity.

Should a priest be called upon to counsel a person in a situation such as application for the use of a kidney machine, about all he can do is to outline the few options presented here. It really comes down to applying and hoping to be selected in which case the priest may be called upon to give a great deal of consolation if the application is denied.

Here we get into a deep and complex field where there is a gap or range of options from what could be called strictly ethical positions to those which would fall under the heading of moral decisions going well beyond the letter of any stated moral law. Throughout the whole field there often is a gap between the humane choice, the morally preferable, which may be in opposition to the former, or the morally superior choice which one can do no more than suggest.

Again, while it is by no means an unfailing rule of thumb, it is fairly safe to say that a good human solution is a good Christian solution, especially in view of incarnational theological perspectives. Nevertheless, the good human solution may be less than the ideal Christian solution. At the same time, the ideal Christian solution is almost always the kind of thing which a man can only make by himself. The extent to which a priest may counsel such action is pretty much a matter of the priest's own conscience, his moral and ethical stances, and his understanding of the person he is counseling.

In the meantime, a great many painful decisions must be made. All that we can do is to continue to stress the value, dignity and even the sacredness of man and the absolute equality of all men, so that these will be considered as fully as possible by those who ultimately must make the choices, especially the choices that must be made under emergency conditions. I would like to be more helpful as would everyone who studies and writes in this field, but the fact remains that the matter as stated is pretty much the way things are.

9. They Treat Horses, Don't They?

Not long ago a horse belonging to a friend of mine got tangled up in the tongue of her house trailer. Before she discovered the situation, the animal, frightened and confused, had managed to injure himself pretty badly. The local veterinarian said there was nothing he could do. Among other things the jaw bone was shattered.

My friend is not the kind of person to give up easily, especially on a horse she likes. He was placed in a trailer and driven a couple of hundred miles to Lansing, Michigan, in the middle of the night. Treatment was begun immediately at one of the best veterinary centers in the country. They told my friend that the necessary treatment and surgery could cost $2,000 or more. She replied that she wanted to do everything she could for the horse but that all she had was $600. They agreed to go ahead with treatment.

It continued over a period of a couple of weeks, and the veterinarians kept my friend informed, at their own expense, of the horse's condition and progress. The outlook was hopeful. However, during the third operation performed in Lansing, the horse died. The people at the veterinary center called my friend and expressed their sympathy. They said that because of the extensive surgery involved they could consider the treatment of the animal as a research project and charge her only for emergency service on the day that the horse was taken there for treatment.

At the same time that I shared my friend's grief over the loss of her horse which was little more than a year old, I found myself wondering how many people would have been treated with as much consideration and handled as delicately in figuring out the economics of the matter. It is unfortunate, but I remember all too well cases where heads of families died due to surgical error and the families came home from the funeral to face a mountain of medical bills including, of course, the surgeon's full fee. This is not to say I think there should be no charge whenever a patient dies, but all in all, I think the veterinarians were a little more considerate in the way they approached people and their problems and bills.

As mentioned earlier, the big word now in medical ethics and hospital administration in general is "total patient care." In a way, the Church has spoken pretty consistently in terms of total patient care, insisting that any sick or injured person is entitled to the best of treatment for what ails him, with consideration for his psychological state and careful attention to his spiritual needs. This is echoed in the Bishop's most recent directives. However, the medical profession and health care facility administrators are actually going a step beyond this when they talk to people in the fields of ethics and morality about total patient care.

As mentioned before, everything counts from the time that a patient has to wait in the doctor's office to the way he is treated in the hospital and the way that his financial affairs are handled. Possible services of social workers are considered along with the general relationship of the health care facility and the family of the patient. This raises a great many questions, and all we can do is to tackle them one by one. Let's start with the area most mentioned by those most concerned and who are also doing the most about it. That is the quality of medical care.

It is quite difficult for the professional, let alone the layman, to know what's good and what's bad in a given hospital situation. An out and out inefficient operation is very easy to spot and occasionally there are practices so shoddy that no one is apt to miss them. On the whole, however, most hospitals appear to be clean, brisk and efficient. Hospital personnel are becoming more and more courteous as jobs become scarcer and scarcer. The general management of hospital floors is roughly as efficient as that of most Holiday Inns. Doctors seem to know what they are doing, professionals, paraprofessionals and others come and go with a look of bright, clean, efficient, well-informed, dedicated service about them. All of this can be true in the midst of a situation where patients are actually receiving poor care.

There are many new gadgets, so many new techniques and so many new approaches to so many new things, that one who hasn't been studying the matter right up to the moment, can be confused out of his mind by what is going on in a given hospital at a given moment.

After all, once a patient enters the operating room, only the surgeon and the surgical staff know what really happens. Very few doctors are really sure how accurately laboratory tests are made. They get reports, but rarely do they watch the actual performance of the tests by the technicians who have been known to fake reports on occasions, spill specimens, mix up others and in general render service that would result in a report that could lead to the wrong treatment. This probably isn't any more common than, say, gross traffic errors by bus drivers, but you don't have to smash up too many buses to have a very serious situation.

I can remember an experience of my own, where exhaustive x-ray studies of the gastrointestinal tract "showed" all kinds of conditions which called for all kinds of treatment only to learn that the actual difficulty was in the esophagus.

And then there is always the kind of situation where the treatment is rendered quite properly for one condition while a second condition is ignored. This can result in death or a serious setback for the patient. Beyond that, as already indicated, there is the problem of treatment, and especially operations, that are unnecessary in the first place. None of the things we are talking about here could be called new. Perhaps the reason that it seems to be such a glaring problem in so many places now, is that hospitals are terribly busy places dealing with a tremendous number of people, and that the factors of human error are often at the danger point long before anyone realizes it.

The whole matter of cost would be the subject of a screamingly funny comedy if it weren't for the fact that it results in out and out tragedy for so many people. As recognized for a long time, one serious illness is enough to wipe out just about any family. This becomes even more so as insurance companies tend more and more to deny claims, attempt partial settlement or delay settlement to the point where a sick person is seriously burdened with problems he doesn't need.

As in all other areas we have been discussing, the thing gets terribly complex. It's not easy to point the finger at any one person or department and say the fault lies there. We'll consider economic factors in other portions of this book. Here we will limit our discussion to their relationship to quality medical care.

Of course, horses aren't people, but the kind of treatment that my friend's horse had in Lansing involved a great deal of skill by a great many specialists, all kinds of tests and special procedures—in short, they would have been expensive by any standard. Still, the most that the veterinary center was talking about was a couple of thousand dollars, which would have included a couple of operations and an indefinite stay for the injured horse.

Without any surgery at all, in fact without much of anything, my son ran up $600 in hospital and medical bills in three days not long ago. That's the same amount that the veterinarians settled for when my friend explained that was all the money she had. Again, I know people will say horses are not humans and their treatment is different. That doesn't necessarily mean that it is that much cheaper.

One of the factors that makes costs so high is closely related to quality of medical practice. Naturally, when a physician is presented with a case when there is some question of diagnosis, he will rely on all kinds of laboratory and x-ray studies in an effort to be as accurate as possible in determining what is wrong and how wrong it is. That is quite understandable.

However, in many cases, a good history and physical, backed up by carefully chosen laboratory and x-ray procedures would be sufficient to establish diagnosis. A more common practice is to admit the patient to the hospital and order every test known to God and man. When they are all completed, the physician still has the task of deciding what is wrong. Many of the tests ordered routinely upon admission have little or no bearing on the matter at hand.

A great many physicians and surgeons have standing orders in hospitals calling for certain procedures to be performed on every patient admitted. In a way it's a precautionary measure, but largely it's a matter of saving time for the physician who would otherwise have to decide exactly what tests were needed and order these individually for patients.

Much the same thing is true in the case of routine medication. Standing orders are left and the patient quite often receives various medications whether he needs them or not. Every single one of these items is carefully noted and sent through an elaborate accounting system which helps to explain why the bill is as high as it is when the patient finally recovers and goes home.

Practically every move made in any direction within a hospital results in a charge slip of some kind being made out. For instance, a patient who is admitted for routine surgery can figure on a fair amount of medicine, all of which will be very costly. If he is admitted through the emergency room, he will pay a charge for the use of that, as well as for any supplies used while he was there. For the operating room he pays a basic charge which goes up if the operation runs any length of time. Then there is a fee for the anesthetist or anesthesiologist and more charge for any special equipment or special studies used in the course of the surgery. Postoperative medications will be another item on the bill as will any rehabilitative procedures which may be ordered.

The point I am trying to make is that costs being what they are, the patient has the right to expect that only those tests, procedures and medications which are necessary for the best treatment of his condition be ordered and charged to him. Going at it any other way is unethical not only economically but also from the point of view that the patient may be subjected to unnecessary inconvenience and pain and may even receive medication which is harmful.

Mark well, we are referring to cases where doctors operate pretty much on standing orders, making very few variations in individual cases. Even when they *do* make these variations, the standing orders are sometimes carried out anyway.

The burden here is pretty much on the physician. Unless he orders something which is absolutely out of line and someone questions it on the grounds of possible danger to the patient, whatever he orders will be done and duly charged for. Rarely if ever does he directly profit from this. The money goes to the hospital. His profit, in addition to whatever fee he may receive for performing an operation, comes from visits to the patient. With rare exceptions, these last from 5 seconds to 5 minutes, and the doctor's office bills so many dollars per visit regardless of its length or what may have been involved. A charge of $15 per visit is not unusual in some places and $15 is a lot for thirty seconds worth of routine conversation which is often what the visit consists of.

Most doctors' visits in hospitals are so hurried that the patient rarely gets to ask questions that he has waited all day to ask. No one else is allowed to answer these questions. Patients have been known to spend several extra days in the hospital because their doctors did not get around to discharging them.

There are areas where the ethics of the hospital have to be considered, too. Hospitals are notoriously wasteful of materials and their losses due to pilferage are frequently extreme. This is reflected in the charge to the patient. Hospitals "cry poor mouth" more than any other kind of institution I can think of. If you really took them seriously, you would get the impression that they were all going out of business tomorrow unless someone gives them several million dollars right now. In plain fact, I know of more than one "non-profit" hospital that operates at a rather tidy profit.

One of the worst causes of the continuing high cost of hospital care is an obsession with purchasing every new diagnostic and therapeutic tool, device or gadget that appears on the market. In some places there is actually a kind of competition in the purchase of these which amounts to keeping up with the Joneses. On the other hand, patients hear about these things and expect their hospitals to have them. In many cases the machinery involved could be done without. It is invariably expensive and the expense is invariably borne by the patient. One would have to weigh the ethical status of each individual purchase, but it would certainly do no harm to warn hospital administrators that there is more involved in health care than simply having all the latest machines.

Much of what we have been discussing here also applies to private doctors' offices or group practice clinics. One physician I know says that until we reach a point in private practice where procedures are not tied to fees and fees to procedures there can be no hope of coming anywhere near a legitimate bill for the patient. In other words, the patient pays so much for an office visit. He also pays so much for a lab test, he also pays for an injection he may not need and so much for each of several other things which he may or may not need. He can easily run up a $25 to $50 bill in less than an hour. That is less than an hour after he completed waiting an hour or two to get in in the first place.

What my friend is saying is that for the most part a flat fee for an office call would be more than sufficient. It might also encourage physicians to avoid unnecessary tests and medications. I have known of many who gave vitamin shots routinely at substantial cost to the patient when there was no possible way to argue that these would be any more beneficial than vitamin tablets taken out of a bottle bought at any drug store. In fact the vitamins probably could have been skipped completely. The fee-for-procedure-approach is well locked into the profession. Just how ethical it is in the practice of each individual physician, only he or some board of inquiry can decide, but occasionally it gets out of hand to the point of being criminal.

I recall a case in New York where a "society doctor" used to give most of his hospital patients blood transfusions. Although starting a blood transfusion is a fairly routine procedure, he used to perform it himself for a fee of $15. The actual work involved by the physician would not take more than five minutes. So attached was this particular doctor to the blood transfusion procedure, that he gave one to a man suffering from high blood pressure. The patient died. The doctor collected his $15.

It might strike you at this point that we are lapsing

from serious consideration of ethical and moral matters into a medical exposé or an attack on the medical profession. This is far from the truth. In the first place, ethics and morality are clearly involved here and the matters referred to are common enough that any physician can afford a few minutes to examine his conscience. The same can be said of administrators of many hospitals.

The ethical physician can be expected to use all of the knowledge and skill at his command to arrive at an accurate diagnosis in the shortest time in the most economical manner possible. An ethical surgeon can be expected to perform only that surgery which is clearly indicated by clinical studies in the most skillful manner of which he is capable, with absolute minimum risk to the patient. He is also ethically responsible to know something about the patient before the operation and to pay some attention to the patient after the operation. In cases where the patient is referred to the surgeon, this foreknowledge and afterknowledge is often casual or all but nonexistent.

The surgeon's responsibility does not begin and end in the operating room. He has a definite ethical obligation to determine if the requested surgery should be done in the first place. He has a definite ethical responsibility to determine what variables and what risks may exist in a given case. He has a definite ethical obligation to be in the best possible condition to perform the surgery and to perform it in the most serious and efficient manner he can. He has a further definite ethical obligation to follow up on the patient until he is sure no risks remain and that recovery is virtually certain, given routine care and allowing for legitimate unforeseen complications. Anything less cannot be called legitimate practice.

Hospitals have a definite ethical obligation to make sure that this kind of practice is conducted routinely by each and every member of the staff. A member who errs too frequently, who is negligent too frequently or who shows definite lack of skill in practice should be barred from further practice in the hospital. Very often such actions are not taken until some serious error has occurred. The busy atmosphere of the hospital can be blamed to some extent. However, it is regrettable that it usually takes the threat of a heavy lawsuit to make most hospitals take definite action to straighten out an offending physician or surgeon.

A terribly serious matter referred to frequently by those who are interested in the quality of medical care is the overdrugging of patients. There are no responsible figures available, but anyone familiar with the matter can tell you that a very heavy percentage of women who go to physicians' offices come out with a prescription for some kind of tranquilizer or sedative. Matter of fact, the male-female difference may not be that great. In addition to the rather high cost of such medication, there is the plain fact that we have developed an extremely drug conscious population as a result of this kind of practice.

It is terribly easy for just about anyone to obtain just about any combination of drugs if he shops around a little in doctors' offices. Many doctors will prescribe drugs at the drop of a hat, sometimes with little more reason than the fact that the retail man visited him that day and suggested that a given drug might be helpful in certain cases. The doctor can get rid of his less sick and more annoying patients rather easily by means of this kind of prescription and probably there is little harm done in occasionally giving someone a tranquilizer or sedative.

The truth is, though, that there are a great many people at large in our society who regulate almost their every physiological function with one drug or another, and they could not do so without the rather careless cooperation of some members of the medical profession. The extent to which drug dependency is physical or purely psychological is questionable from case to case, but it is quite likely that some of the worst offenders in the tranquilizer field could be aided in other ways or could get along without the tranquilizers altogether.

There are other cases, where fairly regular taking of calming drugs of one kind or another may actually hold off more serious conditions ranging from physical illness to psychosis. The medical judgments involved in prescribing in such cases are terribly complicated and no physician should be automatically blamed if he supplies a given patient with what seems to be a rather heavy supply of drugs. The only ethical criterion would seem to be that no drug should be given to any patient unless he needs it and that he should never be given more than he needs to handle a given situation. Here again, there are variables. Judgments have to be presumed to be in good faith until there is rather clear evidence that someone is being careless somewhere.

It certainly is not the task of the priest to encourage patients to question and doubt the competence of their physicians. On the other hand there seems to be a clear pastoral obligation to keep people aware of the moral questions involved in the excessive use of drugs. No one can say for sure how many traffic and industrial accidents result from drugs, often taken unnecessarily. No one can say what serious psychological conditions may result from prolonged drug taking.

This much is so: taking drugs in various combinations, unless carefully supervised, can lead to bad psychological effects and sometimes bad physiological effects as well. The effects may even be fatal.

The ethical weight falls on both the physician and patient. The patient should be able to assume that he will not be given drugs other than those he needs in the amount he needs in a given situation. If a client for pastoral counseling is clearly reliant on drugs and there is reason to believe that drug dependency could be overcome, then there are rather distinct moral questions. It is a general presumption that one has an obligation to face reality as clearly and sharply as possible. The constant avoiding of it—by the use of alcohol or drugs is certainly not in the best interest of anyone's moral and spiritual development.

A clearly questionable practice in some hospitals, particularly in psychiatric sections, is the routine over-drugging of annoying or troublesome patients.

Drugging a patient merely to make him "more co-operative" is not apt to contribute very much to his recovery. In some state hospitals, there has been suspicion more than once that patients actually died as a result of excessive drugging, sometimes carried out in combination with having them sleep in cold, overly ventilated quarters. Many of the cases under suspicion involved the excessive use of Phenobarbital, since Phenobarbital poisoning produces symptoms much like hypostatic pneumonia. No one will ever know how many "pneumonia deaths" in certain state hospitals had little to do with pneumonia itself.

This chapter provides only a quick look into the overall field of poor patient care, but it should give you some idea of just what is involved. In chapters to follow, we will point out some other areas, perhaps not as immediately damaging to patients, but just as serious to anyone who is concerned with total patient care of high quality.

10. Everyman Goes
to the Hospital

Continuing the business of discussing total patient care as an ethical and moral goal of the health care professions and the facilities in which they function, we are, with some apology, going to have to introduce even more confusion. There is so much involved, that we may not even refer specifically to ethical or moral issues.

Because we are concerned with the entire man and his welfare, everything we talk about has ethical or moral implications and we'll only point out the big questions. As in so much of the material already covered, there is a terrible lack of answers. The most we can strive for is openness, understanding, and the development of the kind of attitudes and judgments that will make the ordinary priest in the ordinary medical situation a good and wise counselor. It's a long time since I've used the term "grace of state" but if you still believe in that sort of thing you might be very grateful for it. That alone may lead to answers which everybody is finding hard to come by.

Recall that we are dealing with improved quality of care in relation to the concept of total patient care. We have broadened our whole base and have taken a specific direction. Mere progress is not enough. Improved quality is mandatory. At the same time that efforts are being made to achieve that, countless new situations arise and have to be fit into the context of total patient care while their quality is evaluated and efforts are made to improve it where it is lacking.

Throughout the writing of a chapter like this, I have to exercise particular self-control, because I've been associated one way or another with hospitals since I was 16 years old and was hanging around pathology labs, come to think of it, a couple of years before that. To further complicate the matter I was passionately interested in genetics at about the age of 12. The changes that I observed, I'm now 48, are simply beyond belief. I thought I saw a medical revolution during and just following World War II. That of course was a mild development compared to what has happened since.

For instance, within my own lifetime, there were still a great many people who considered a hospital as a place you went to die. I took ambulance calls out of a hospital in a predominantly Italian district while I was a student and remember clearly that you very often had to talk older Italian people into getting on the stretcher and leaving their homes to go to the hospital. Someone often covered the face of the patient to spare him taking his last look at the house and the crowd surrounding the ambulance. A procession of relatives and friends usually followed the stretcher to the ambulance weeping and wailing, apparently convinced that they had seen the last of a loved one. Unfortunately this was true more often than not, because the loved ones usually waited until it was too late to go to the hospital.

During those years and years that followed, I saw

a lot of emergency situations handled on the street not only by ambulance crews but by fire and police department rescue squads. All of this shakes me up just a little bit when I watch a TV program like "Emergency" based on paramedics being used in the field in a major metropolitan area. There is a distinct trend toward the use of these people, and, for the most part, it seems to be a good one, but let me point out where some of the personal difficulty comes in.

I am old enough to remember when a young M.D. rode the ambulance on all but the most routine calls and sometimes even on those. These interns had a full medical education and had picked up at least some practical experience along the way. Presumably, this was superior to what anyone could give a paramedic in a crash course or even in an extended course. The fact is, the intern usually got a great deal of advice from the ambulance driver on how to handle the situation on the street, whether it was an accident with a lot of fractures and severe lacerations, an obstetrical case or a heart attack.

The young doctor was not trained for medicine in the field to any great extent and the ambulance driver, although he might lack even a high school education, had simply been around long enough that he could often reduce a compound fracture on the spot with considerable skill, deliver babies with little difficulty and follow with pretty sure instinct and considerable ability whatever procedures were necessary to prepare the patient for transportation and to get him to the hospital safely.

The general idea was to avoid or minimize shock, immobilize fractures and suspected fractures, avoid injury to the patient in the way he was placed on the stretcher and carried in the ambulance, use oxygen if necessary and in extreme cases administer adrenalin or coramine. There was no particular attempt to "stabilize" the condition of the patient before he was moved. The general policy was to take care of things that obviously had to be taken care of on the spot and get him to the hospital as quickly as possible so the real treatment could begin.

In fact, for a long time, individual doctors and professional associations made quite a point of saying that there was no point in rushing most people to the hospital, that a safe, reasonably quick ride was all that was required and that very little was saved by excessive speed in transportation.

The thesis of the paramedic field crew today seems to be that insofar as possible the condition should be stabilized before transportation and this, if you want to go by the kind of procedures indicated on the TV show referred to, can often consist of considerable time spent starting infusions or transfusions, dealing with cardiac symptoms and taking various other measures before transportation is begun. The paramedic is advised by radio or telephone of the proper steps to take after he reports the condition of the patient in some detail from the scene.

Operations like this are in progress in many places, although they probably lack some of the more advanced equipment shown on TV and certainly don't constantly run into all of the highly critical situations that the program presents. The point is, there is a great deal of training of ambulance personnel going on. More and more responsibility, previously considered the exclusive domain of the doctor and only practiced in his absence under the most extreme circumstances, is now routinely handled by paramedics more or less under supervision.

This really shouldn't shock anyone, since the armed forces have had to make use of highly trained paramedics for a long time in order to provide anything like adequate medical service in the field. Many of these same men are involved in the paramedic programs being set up now in some of our major cities. A great many have a good background, quite a bit of experience and a great deal of skill. As in anything else, however, the courses a man has taken and the experience he has had don't actually guarantee much of anything. There are medics and then there are medics in any branch of the armed forces. Some may have performed highly advanced procedures, while others have done little more than orderly work or have given shots to men standing in a line.

Further, these men are now dealing with civilian situations and civilian patients have considerably more in the way of immediate rights and legal protection than a battlefield casualty who is usually more than happy to settle for the services of anyone who comes along with anything looking like medical aid.

Frankly, I am a little bit frightened of the situation while admitting that it is probably basically good and in the long run will probably fill needs that otherwise would go unfilled. One of the big things that brought about the change of philosophy was a rather radical development in the handling of cardiac patients who can "be brought back to life" by some of our more recent equipment. Obviously, the term "brought back to life" is not a correct one, even though it is used rather commonly by some doctors. Nevertheless, a man's life presumably may be saved instantly on the street, whereby it might have been lost had old-time procedures been used.

In actuality, I can't help wondering how many times this is really so. As I remember cardiac patients in emergency call situations, they were either obviously dead upon arrival of the ambulance or else they survived the trip to the hospital with the aid of a little oxygen and perhaps a stimulant. If they managed that, they had a fairly good chance of recovery. I even wonder how much difference the starting of an infusion at the scene makes when the patient will probably be in the hospital within a matter of minutes. Infusions and transfusions are not that difficult to start, but they do carry with them a certain risk of error and some of the errors can be fatal.

In other words, I would like to see them carried out under maximum supervision, even though a person may actually perform them with a little training and good direction.

What is done now in the intensive care units and special cardiac sections of our better hospitals borders on the miraculous. No one is going to quarrel with that. Whether this dictates extending these procedures to the street and whether that extension actually has any wholesale benefits is another question. I won't try to answer it.

One case where it might be of distinct help is in rural and semirural situations where the transportation time is considerably more than it would be within a city. Here there might be some great benefit in stabilizing conditions before transportation and it is possible that lives might be saved on the spot when the patient could not otherwise last long enough to get to the hospital. But rather critical judgments are involved and in the rural and semirural situation the ability to get firsthand advice from a highly qualified physician may be severely restricted. A great many of the hospitals serving these areas don't have a physician present during night-time hours. One has to be called in. The time a man qualified to give instructions on complicated cardiac care might be reached and put in touch with an ambulance crew on the scene might very well balance off any benefits to be gained from delaying transportation of the patient. Leaving the kind of judgments involved in the hands of an ambulance crew, no matter how well trained, is, I guess, just a little bit too "progressive" a measure for me to be able to swallow at the present time.

I don't mind telling you why. Less than a year ago I came upon an accident victim only minutes after the crash. He was driving. The passengers were not badly injured and were flagging down cars to get aid in a very remote place, at least 40 minutes from the nearest ambulance. Having rather clear-cut signs that the man was about as close to death as you can get, and that any measures were probably better than none, I sent one of the less injured passengers in my car to call for police and an ambulance and did the best I could on an icy road to employ external heart massage and mouth-to-mouth resuscitation. It was successful, and the victim was talking with me and a little bit with his wife by the time the ambulance arrived.

It was a small town rescue squad unit manned by two men, members of a group which had undergone extensive training over a long period of time. They had great difficulty even getting the man onto the stretcher properly and then put it in the ambulance backwards.

I believe I stopped for a drink before going home. Fortunately, the patient survived.

I can justify my own actions by saying that no other help was immediately available, that the situation was obviously critical and that my action probably was better than none under the circumstances, since I did know what I was doing. I can't help wondering, though, how such a situation would be handled by a crew that can't even figure out which end of the stretcher goes into the ambulance first.

Another rather alarming aspect of this situation came up not too long ago when some recent graduates of an emergency medical technician program in a community college went to work in a hospital in a small city as combination orderlies and ambulance attendants. They had received a great deal of training, and apparently it was good training, in all kinds of emergency procedures, including tracheotomies.[1] I became aware that one of the young men was just itching for his first opportunity to perform a tracheotomy in the field. I know few highly qualified medical people who are in any hurry to do that and I am particularly happy that the young man in question never got near my own trachea. As far as I know the hospital calmed him down before he decided to try brain surgery on the street, but this case, which is not an isolated one by any means, does suggest that while paramedics of all kinds will undoubtedly be needed to keep health care facilities running, something more than training courses and remote supervision may be necessary if the patient is to get safe, high quality care.

The same kind of thing happens within hospitals.

---

[1] Cutting into the "windpipe" when the breathing passage is blocked or otherwise disabled.

Shortages in all fields being what they are where health care is concerned, graduates of various short-term courses or training programs conducted within the hospitals themselves are used to perform rather complicated procedures. For the most part, this is to the patient's benefit, assuming that a reasonable selection of personnel was made. The personnel involved are very carefully limited to the precise procedures for which they were trained and their performance is periodically evaluated. The difficulty is that, in both large and small hospitals, supervision and evaluation are often difficult. All kinds of things and people seem to get lost in big medical centers and smaller places get so chummy and so busy at the same time, that almost anything can happen.

For example, the great increase in the use of practical or vocational nurses, generally graduates of one-year programs, has been a great boon to hospitals who could not find a sufficient number of registered nurses to perform all of the work that needed to be done. Nurses' aides generally lack the educational background and direct experience to perform these functions well. So the practical nurse came into her own, but not without some problems.

Many smaller hospitals, hospitals in rural and semi-rural communities and extended care facilities in urban areas often use a maximum number of practical nurses and a minimum number of registered nurses for purely economic reasons. The practical nurse usually gets at least a dollar an hour less than a registered nurse. This means that the R.N. is pretty much desk-bound, limited to supervisory functions and the keeping of records, although the latter may be delegated to a ward secretary to some extent.

In all, that's not a bad setup, but it does lead to difficulties. In some places practical nurses with several years of experience, particularly in some specialized areas, actually manage to rule over registered nurses and perform functions which even registered nurses would rarely attempt.

The most shocking example I can think of, in a fully accredited hospital, is the case of a practical nurse who very frequently performs episiotomies[2] on obstetrical patients during night-time deliveries when doctors are a little slow to get to the scene.

To date she has had no real difficulty that I know of, but the legal risks inherent in the situation are awful to say the least and it is very unlikely that the patient came to the hospital with the idea of having a practical nurse perform any surgical procedure on her.

Most deliveries come off pretty routinely, but the occasional one that doesn't calls for instant decisions, instant actions and provides an extremely narrow margin for error if mother and infant are to survive. Having a delivery room presided over by a practical nurse doesn't seem to be the best possible way to be prepared for these occasional, but very real cases.

The hospitals involved can't possibly have house staffs. The doctors involved can't possibly stay at the hospital twenty-four hours a day. It does seem, though, that they could anticipate their deliveries a little bit better, although this is by no means the easiest thing to do, and could make every effort to get to the hospital a little bit quicker. Many have been known to refuse to come in at night at all. Here there is very little room for argument as to the ethics of the situation.

Even the so called "professionalization" of nurses

---

[2] Widening the birth canal by incising the perineum.

has not been an unmixed blessing. I remember, some-what fondly, when girls entering nursing school spent their first six months as "probies," generally wearing black stockings, black shoes and a slightly frightened and highly respectful expression. They held doors for doctors and called practically everybody "sir." They did the most menial work on the wards, including scrubbing floors. At the same time, they got their intro-ductory classwork and a pretty good notion of what goes on in a hospital. At the end of these early tor-turous months, they got white stockings and shoes and before long, student nurses' caps.

By this time, they were really quite handy. They usually worked regular shifts, assisting graduate person-nel in patient care under close supervision. It was a tough life. Often they worked all night and had to man-age to stay up for their classes during the daytime, then get enough rest to go back to work for another night. During a three-year period they rotated pretty well through the hospital and were exposed to all of the usual functions of a general health care facility. If a special kind of care was not offered in the hospital where they trained, they were sent elsewhere for "affili-ation" in fields such as psychiatry and care of tuber-cular patients.

By the time these girls were in their third year of training, they were very close to being capable of taking over a floor for a short period of time and in an emer-gency for an entire shift. By the last half of their third year, there was little doubt of their competence. Any-one who had lasted through the grind that they had simply had to have something on the ball. Some were better than others, but I remember them all rather fondly and with considerable respect.

A graduate of such a program could go into just about any hospital and with a minimum of orientation and perhaps a little specialized additional training, become adept at providing good patient care wherever it was needed. Some went on and specialized to a larger extent and became extremely capable people. A small percentage went into administration.

Then came "professionalization" and the proliferation of degree programs in nursing where a large share of the work was done on a college campus and clinical experience was considerably reduced. Often the student nurse was on the floor only as an observer. Her total clinical experience at the end of her education was considerably less than that of the old three-year graduate no matter what anyone says.

Also, old-time hospital workers will tell you that often these girls just don't have it where practical things are involved. They have a somewhat inflated opinion of themselves based on the fact that they go into their jobs as college graduates and "professionals" (nursing was always considered a profession in modern times) but often don't know the first thing about some of the essentials of keeping a floor running.

The most hilarious example I know happened when a college senior in a nursing program was in her sister's home when the baby became sick. The sister called a doctor who asked to have a rectal temperature taken. The fourth-year student, near-professional, did not have the slightest idea of how to go about the procedure. This may seem like an exaggeration, but I can swear to every detail. It happened in my own family.

Then entered another whole species to further complicate the health care scene. Again, it was almost certainly necessary, but not an unmixed blessing. This is the species administrator. Hospitals have always needed superintendents or administrators and these always needed assistants who presided over a corps of clerks who handled things like admitting of patients, bookkeeping, and the overseeing of various departments such as housekeeping and food services.

Professional training of hospital administrators in large universities is by no means a new development. However, their number has increased considerably and they seem to be rather a different breed. The old timer, and here I am referring to someone who would have been functioning in the forties and early fifties, was in many cases a physician. Sometimes the administrator was a nurse. I have known others who were pharmacists who took graduate training in hospital administration. Others had a business administration background. They were a kind of minority within a hospital, in spite of their obvious importance. With the exception of the top man, however, they were generally regarded with a little disdain by people who worked on the patient care end of things. Then, just as in education, the species administrator became unbelievably numerous, unbelievably complicated and unbelievably hard to live with.

By now we have personnel men, accountants, computer men, purchasing experts, P.R. men, any conceivable variety of people with non-medical skills who are brought into the running of a hospital because of its increasingly complex nature. Now don't get me wrong, these people are needed. However, at the upper levels, they follow a rule in practice which can be observed in many commercial endeavors and certainly in most educational institutions. They are committee-oriented, terribly threatened in general and could be

described in many cases as work causers, work con-
fusers, work losers, work observers, work changers,
and work thinker-uppers. That adds up to a lot of
work which invariably has to be done by someone else.
Finding that someone else is often a problem well
beyond the capabilities of the administrative corps.

Of course, there are notable exceptions, near-geni-
uses who have made fantastic contributions to the
health care field. Unfortunately, they are not easy
to find.

Now I have gone into all of this detail to give you
some of the darker side of what appears to be a very
bright, efficient, hustling up-to-the-minute operation
that Everyman encounters when he enters a hospital,
whether he has been zapped by the paramedics in advance or not. The possibilities of human errors which
directly affect the patient are equally immense. The
possibilities of confused records, medication errors and
other disasters and near disasters are something that no
one likes to contemplate.

At another level, unnecessary suffering may result
from poor functions of a health care facility, not to
mention unnecessary expense, plain inconvenience and
a kind of frustration that can only be known to one who
has had to spend quite a bit of time in hospitals. Don't
be too sure that the gripes you hear from a patient you
visit are a result of some neurosis of his. He may in
fact have witnessed unbelievable scenes and have been
the victim of unbelievable situations.

Of course the head nurse, like the proper school
teacher, manages to write off most of these things by
saying that the patient, like the complaining student,
has a "bad attitude" or is "uncooperative." On the sur-
face it would seem that the patient in today's hospital

is getting the best care possible, care far superior to that given in past years. In fact, he may be benefitting from better medical care, although that is not a certainty, but it is very doubtful that the service he is getting is that much improved, even though there may be the appearance of efficiency that we have referred to often.

Bureaucrats tend to arrange things so that a maximum number of personnel is available when the bureaucrats actually have to function. That means during rather normal business hours. That, in turn, means that you will find a proliferation of personnel on the floors of many hospitals on the day shift that is astounding to contemplate. They literally trip over each other in many instances. Their numbers thin out considerably as the afternoon shift takes over and by the time the night shift comes to work, the floor on which Everyman gets his treatment may be a very lonely place in terms of personnel.

Of course, there is some reason for this. Most treatments are given during the daytime and there is less need for personnel on the night shift than on the evening shift. But the differences in assignment often are out of proportion. Evening shifts admit most patients who come in for things like elective surgery and this is a fairly time-consuming procedure. They still have medications to give and visitors to handle as well as a lot of patients who are having trouble getting to sleep. In general, it has always been a difficult shift.

Things are a little quieter for the night shift—only treatments which are absolutely necessary, only medications which must be given at regular intervals even during the night, and in general a somewhat more subdued situation. However, some of the very worst situations occur at night, often without warning, and emergencies have a habit of coming in while the night shift carries the ball. This is when their limited numbers become a real problem in some hospitals.

Everyman will gain something from today's hospital management. He will generally get to select his meals a day in advance and they tend to be a little bit better than the food served in hospitals a few years back. That isn't to say that they're good, just better. He will be treated with a reasonable amount of courtesy by hospital personnel, but there is a thin line between human concern and compassion, courtesy and what we might call the "airline treatment." A certain amount of the bright and sunny disposition of the airline stewardess or ticket agent can be found in many hospitals where the administration has decided that things have to be more cheerful and the morale of patients has to be kept at a higher level. Nothing is apt to decrease morale so much as a phony smile and an overly solicitous manner. Ask Everyman the fourth day after he has been in the hospital for treatment of, say, an ulcer.

One of the sharpest hospital administrators I know[3] made a painful observation to me not long ago. She pointed out that patients used to feel neglected and used to lie in their beds for long hours with little conversation and little to look forward to except visiting hours and meal times. "Now," she said, "the patient is apt to be visited by a freshman medical student, a sophomore medical student, a junior medical student, a senior medical student, an intern, an assistant resident, a resident, a student practical nurse, a student nurse, a psychologist "interning" in the hospital, a social worker, three seminarians, two clergymen, an ombuds-

[3] Sister Mary Janice Belen.

man, and a news vendor in the course of an afternoon. This concern with keeping the patient occupied and reassured is a fine thing. It's good to get students in the health care professions into direct patient contact earlier than they used to. In fact, the whole idea behind the visitation is excellent."

"But what about the poor patient?" she asked. "He probably is supposed to be getting some rest. He undoubtedly would like a little bit of privacy. He certainly must get sick of telling his story over and over again, no matter how much he likes to tell his story."

This administrator is exceptionally candid as well as exceptionally perceptive. We pay a price for progress no matter where or when we achieve it. Our best ideas often degenerate into our worst circumstances.

From a purely ethical and moral standpoint about all that can be said is anytime the practices, procedures and policies of the hospital don't actually result in a higher quality of patient care, the goal is being missed and the patient may be receiving less care than he is entitled to. His personal wishes and general comfort may suffer considerably.

The only thing we can say at this point is: Don't be faked out by the glitter and hurry-scurry.

Some of the finest people in the world work in and around hospitals. Many could make a lot more money doing something else. Of course, some couldn't make a living doing anything else. From the standpoint of a priest visiting in a hospital or serving as a chaplain, what's necessary is an appreciation for what is being done and what the administration is trying to achieve while at the same time retaining a sufficiently jaundiced eye to be aware of real failings that take place in the midst of what appear to be the finest medical facilities.

There are other problems that are mentioned frequently in connection with improvement of total patient care and a general upgrading of the quality of that care. One is the business of discharging patients too soon or moving them to extended care facilities in order to free beds or serve some economic end. Even though it might be an attempt to keep costs down for the patient, too soon is still too soon. On the other side of that coin there is the tendency to keep some patients in the hospital too long, either because of a hyper-cautious attitude or because of the family's insistence that, "Grandma just isn't ready to go home."

A physician has some very difficult choices to make in some of these cases and the thing for the man interested in ethics and morality to be on the lookout for is not so much the instance of poor judgment as the deliberate extended stay or the deliberate stay cut short for economic reasons, for reasons serving only the convenience of the physician, or for reasons involving family pressure which may come from very selfish motives. If one is really wondering as to how ready grandma is to go home, it's often a good idea to ask grandma.

The sad fact is that there are people who like to have other people sick, even need to have them sick. I remember a case in an extended care facility where a man who had been largely bed-ridden for several years was aided to get up and around a little bit and finally was able to wear a pair of pants for the first time in a long time. When his wife visited the institution and found that he was walking and actually had pants on, she was furious. It was hard to tell exactly why she was furious, but apparently she had some need to have him chronically sick with no real hope of returning home. The sight of the poor fellow wearing pants was simply more than she could bear. He enjoyed them immensely.

A great problem, which shows up painfully in hospitals just as in every other phase of American life is racial discrimination. Laws in most states forbid it, most hospitals have policies which forbid it in general, but it is a distinct reality in many, many places. It isn't that long ago that I visited a Catholic hospital in one of the southern states and found that they no longer had a door marked "colored" and another door marked "white." They simply had a door marked "one" and another marked "two."

As in other things, however, all the blame can't be heaped on the South. Delicate little arrangements are often made so that black patients are placed together and every effort is made to spare placing a white woman in a semi-private room with a black woman. It would seem that we should have gotten past that a long time ago. Larger wards have been racially mixed for years and no one has seemed to suffer, but the same prissy little kind of concern with the feelings of the prejudiced white persists to an awful degree.

In most places it could not be said that the black patient receives treatment inferior to the white patient, assuming that he can afford to be in the hospital in the first place and that he can find one with "enough room" to take him. For many blacks these things are simply impossibilities. The discrimination goes right up the ladder. Black nurses are pretty well treated now, but black physicians still find themselves running into considerable prejudice.

One instance noted by Dr. Hellegers[4] and observed

---

[4] During a Conference on the Ethical and Religious Directives for Health Care Facilities, held at Mercy Center, Farmington, Michigan, April 1972.

by many others is that in quite a few hospitals a black resident physician is not allowed to perform a pelvic examination on a white patient. There are hospitals where no house staff member performs pelvic examinations on private patients, but to forbid a man to carry out this procedure simply because he is black seems to be about as bad as discrimination can get. Of course, patients have rights and certain female patients may object to a pelvic examination given by anyone but their own doctors and even raise a litle hell about that. However, anytime that the thing comes down to racial discrimination as a policy of the staff, not reflecting the particular objections of a particular patient, we certainly have an ethical problem.

One thing that may be indicated to the priest thinking in broadly pastoral terms is that the personnel in the hospital may have as much or even more need for his services than the patients. An alert clergyman will often spot such instances and if he is at all open and available they will often be brought directly to him. Some of the most rewarding pastoral experiences come from this kind of case.

If we had to cite some general things that would be of benefit to the priest in the hospital, even when he is not dealing with specifically ethical or moral situations in which he must aid in a decision, it would be that the more perceptive he is, the more willing he is to listen and the more sensibly compassionate he is, the more effective he will be.

One thing more is necessary. Somehow or other, even though it may not come naturally to him, he absolutely has to have a sense of humor. It's like this. He moves in a world where things like the following can happen.

Female patient A is wheeled to surgery for rhinoplasty, (a nose job). Female patient B is wheeled to surgery at the same time for a hemorrhoidectomy. Somehow there is confusion. Female patient A finds her feet in stirrups and certain preparatory measures being taken on her buttocks. Female patient B, quite concerned about her hemmorhoids, finds her nose being painted. It's a world in which one simply has to laugh as well as pray.

11. Confidentiality and Required Examinations

Little needs to be changed in traditional medical ethics and medical morality in these areas. The problem lies not with the ethics but with their lack of use and enforcement. The natural, committed and professional secrets known by everyone in the medical profession are simply not the secrets they used to be. In fact, our whole society suffers from a great lack of personal and corporate privacy and there are few areas where this is more true than in the area of health care.

Again, the difficulty comes largely from the fact that very few people deal with a single physician in the course of their lives. Their histories and records may appear in the offices of many different physicians as well as in many hospitals and other places. Access to these places is by no means strictly limited. Nothing short of a vast overhaul in the entire system seems likely to solve the problem. Even if the system itself were made a lot more foolproof than it is, a great deal needs to be taught to physicians, nurses and paramedical personnel about the importance of the privacy and reputation of an individual human person.

Not long ago, a nurse I know was walking down the street when she ran into the receptionist from an OB-

140

GYN office. The receptionist said: "Oh, you're pregnant already. I'm so glad." The nurse stumbled around for a minute and then asked what in the world she meant. The receptionist said: "Oh, I'm sorry, that must have been your sister that was in the other day." The sister was not married at the time.

Anyone sitting behind a receptionist's desk or making out bills in a doctor's office or clinic comes across a great deal of more or less private information. Strictly speaking, without even getting into secrets, any information provided to a physician's office, clinic or health care facility should be considered private. It is none of anyone's business who goes to what doctor for what and when.

Within a hospital, assuming the job is done correctly, a detailed medical history is taken on each patient and included in his or her chart. This is followed up by progress notes, also made in considerable detail. Presumably, these charts are available only to physicians and nursing personnel. Even they are rather casual at times about discussing information contained therein. However, the situation gets worse than that. In hospitals where controls are rather loosely enforced —and that's a lot of them—practically anyone can get a look at a chart. One guard I know had a habit of passing the long night hours by simply reading through the charts of various patients that he knew. Other hospital personnel have even been known to go into record rooms and dig out charts of former patients to get one or another piece of personal information. It's impossible to find a term that would fully describe the lack of ethics involved.

On the other hand, one of the greatest difficulties that the average hospital has is getting the attending physician to include a good history and to keep his progress notes up-to-date. Either way, everyone seems to be the loser. A good history and good progress notes are absolutely essential; their protection is at least equally essential. Once the patient has been discharged and the records are consigned to the record room as they must be, every precaution should be taken to make sure that they do not fall into unqualified hands.

In practice, "qualified hands" includes an awful lot of hands. By signing up for most hospitalization insurance, the average subscriber gives the insurance company the right to inspect his hospital and medical records anytime that it serves its purpose. Casualty insurance companies representing both the patient and persons with whom he may be involved in litigation may also gain access to the records. A thorough investigator with a few contacts or a good line rarely has any great difficulty finding out the contents of hospital records. If a physician really wants to protect his patients' privacy and reputation, about the only thing he can do is keep certain information out of the files. In so doing, he may actually cause future harm to the patient when someone digs out the records and fails to find information that might be vital in treating some future condition. It would seem that we need laws to restrict the kind and amount of information that may be released for legal purposes. However, the laws themselves would not solve the problem. Laws need to be enforced. Anyone ought to feel perfectly at ease in confiding the most personal and delicate information to a physician. If most people knew how few safeguards there are for this information, they would probably keep a great deal more to themselves than they do. That in turn, could seriously interfere with proper treatment. It's a real dilemma and one that the profession has failed to face squarely.

Few persons realize the harm that is often done to their reputations as a result of the divulging of "privileged information." If such information is traded about in a free and easy manner, a person's job, credit rating, practically any aspect of his life may be affected. The fact that a given person had a venereal disease a few years ago is really nobody's business. The fact that a girl was pregnant outside of marriage is nobody's business except hers and the people immediately concerned with the problem. Yet, such information is readily available to anyone who wants to use a little bit of ingenuity. It may be used against a person in any one of a number of ways.

The more serious a court case is, the more likely it is that someone is going to do a great deal of digging into medical records. Even if the information obtained thereby cannot be used in court, there are many ways of using it against the best interests of the patient. To repeat, privacy is privacy and secrets are secrets. One of the most fundamental teachings of Catholic ethics is that a person has a strict right to his own reputation, even though the reputation be false. The only possible grounds for violating that right would be a waiver by the person himself or a case where the common good was so demanding that there was no choice but to harm a reputation in order to prevent a much greater evil. There are very few such cases.

An area that has bothered me and a few others for a long time but is rarely even considered is that of the required medical examination. The same could be said of required psychological tests and psychiatric evaluations. This is another complex area where flat and easy rules are hard to come by. For instance, a man applying for a job on a police department has to satisfy his prospective employer that he is in good health, agile, emotionally stable, fairly able physically and mentally to meet the demands of his job. The same could be said of fire fighting jobs and many jobs in industry where lack of physical strength, a physical disability or emotional instability could lead to serious injury or death for the person himself or others. In cases like these, there is little doubt that the prospective employer has a right to require a pretty thorough examination.

Persons who are going to handle food or work around the sick should have to satisfy their prospective employers that they are free from communicable disease. However, they are frequently required to undergo examinations which go far beyond that. About the only principle that can be drawn is that no examination should be required of any person that goes beyond the scope of determining his fitness for a particular job. In some cases this will not get very deeply into emotional stability at all. In other cases it will require little more than the information that he has the customary number of feet and hands and can see and hear. There may even be exceptions to these requirements. It could be said in all justice that any prospective employer has a right to know that the person he is considering hiring is in good general health and has reasonable emotional stability. It would seem, however, that such information could be provided by a statement from a reputable physician who is regularly caring for the person. Why an applicant for a routine job should be forced to undergo a complete physical examination by a physician employed by the company is quite a question if you stop and consider it a little. Why he should have to reveal any particular phase of his mental and emotional makeup is likewise questionable. After all, his employment record, references and general life history should be sufficient to satisfy the knowledge that the ordinary employer has the right to expect.

It is true that a family physician may sometimes offer a statement of health that is somewhat prejudiced in favor of the prospective employee. However, this is easily offset by a tendency of some company doctors to be overly strict or overly casual. Yet, the best argument against the practice of wholesale complete physical examinations and psychological evaluations is the readily observable failure to obtain desired results. Probably no group is examined more frequently and thoroughly than nurses and schoolteachers. If you are at all familiar with the health and psychological problems of nurses and schoolteachers, you can see that the examinations don't always do their job too well.

Privacy of person is a matter that has been lost in our society. There is really no reason why a job applicant should have to undress, be examined from head to foot and answer all kinds of personal questions. The only alternative that most applicants have is to withdraw application for the job. If the employer requires it and the prospective employee refuses it, that pretty much ends the matter.

Of course life insurance companies have a certain right to evaluate the risks they are taking by insuring various persons. However, the average insurance examination is so casual that the business of examining for insurance companies is little more than a racket in many cases. On the other hand, the personal investigation conducted regarding the applicant may go far beyond proper bounds of inquiry in proportion to needed information.

Personally, I won't even tell anyone over the phone what I do for a living or what my office address is or even what my name is until I am thoroughly satisfied that I know the identity of the other party and his reason for requesting information. Persons visiting my office and asking questions of any kind for any reason will usually wind up answering more questions than they ask before they get my middle initial. The most extreme case I know was when a recently appointed agent in charge of an FBI office was called by a newspaper and asked for his middle initial. He asked: "For what purpose?" I don't blame him.

It wasn't too many years ago that I gave some rather confidential information to a highly reputable physician. I was somewhat dismayed to find it being discussed freely and happily by his wife and a group of her friends on a country club veranda over luncheon.

The required examination and evaluation has, of course, extended very deeply into our educational system. It's impossible to enroll in most schools without undergoing some kind of examination. Again, the school has a right to know if it is accepting someone who has a particular health problem that needs watching and that it is not enrolling a psychotic. Beyond that, the rights of a school to demand any particular physical or psychological information would seem to very limited. The practice of requiring annual physical examinations of students is another matter which has caused me to raise my eyebrows for many years. In more than one instance the main reason for having it done was to give some medical students an opportunity to get some practice performing examinations. That would hardly seem to be a justifying cause.

Actually, the matter of psychological evaluation is a lot trickier than the procedure of requiring a physical examination, even though the physical examination may involve more embarrassment and discomfort. Examinations that call for manifestation of conscience in any form by the person being psychologically evaluated are certainly out of line unless the person is clearly informed of what is going on and freely consents to the manifestation of conscience. On the whole, the psychological profession just doesn't see it this way. They feel that the examiner is entitled to ask anything and get a reasonably accurate answer. I heard of a particularly lovely case recently where a western seminary has employed a female psychiatrist to interview and work with all students. The first question she asks most seminarians is: "What is your sex life like?"

Again, the student often has very little choice. Certain tests and examinations are required for admission and his refusal to take one or more may lead to a refusal to admit him to the institution of his choice. Certainly, a seminary or religious order has a right to know if an applicant is healthy and reasonably sane. It would seem, however, that many seminaries and religious orders as well as general academic institutions are out of bounds. This is particularly true in the case of a person who is already a student and who may be required to take psychological testing or undergo a psychological interview. I have known of cases in seminaries and religious orders where the only alternative was to withdraw. It seems to me that this is both unfair coercion and a violation of privacy. It generally follows some disciplinary matter and it would seem that the ethical course is to treat the disciplinary matter as such, not to probe beyond reason into the consciousness or subconscious of the subject.

A great deal of difficulty in psychological testing lies with the interpretation of the examiner. The test itself may be a reasonably good one, but an examiner, having given a battery of tests, generally summarizes his findings and offers an opinion. This is about as unscientific as you can get. The tests themselves have certain built-in "guarantees" of reliability and validity, but even the most careful opinion of the most cautious examiner leaves us a long way from certitude and could, intentionally or not, lead to a very unfair judgment against the subject.

There is a further problem which neither the medical profession nor the psychological profession has any real control over and that is the use made by those who receive the results of the examination. A doctor examining a prospective employee may feel that he is perfectly healthy enough for the job in question, but his report may be used in a way which would cause a particular applicant to be rejected. The same thing could certainly be true of paying too much attention to the results of psychological or psychiatric evaluations. I can testify to more than one instance where a person was said to be hopelessly psychotic by a highly qualified practitioner. The persons involved are moving about freely and living perfectly good, healthy lives today. Similarly, practically everyone knows of people who were told that they were going to die within six months or that they would never walk again. The persons in many cases are still alive and walking quite nicely.

Given any choice in the matter, I believe an employer or administrator should require a statement of health consistent with the demands of the job or the conditions of the educational institution. Periodic review of these would not be out of order. The important principle seems to be to limit examinations and evaluations to those that are absolutely necessary to provide information which is absolutely necessary for the best possible conduct of a business or institution. In all cases, if examinations and evaluations are required, they should be paid for by the requiring agency. A number of years ago I ran into a case where a Catholic hospital in Texas required all personnel to have exhaustive physical examinations at their own expense. This strikes me as being unjust on the face of it and, in addition, could open the door to some genuinely unscrupulous conduct in requiring all kinds of things that employees would have to pay for as conditions of continued employment. It would be very hard to argue that this is in any way ethical.

As for psychological evaluation, as valuable as it can be under some circumstances, persons requiring it should give some thought to an applicant's past record and to a considered evaluation of an employee's or student's performance by competent persons in positions to observe this.

In one recent academic situation we met weekly, a staff of four, and reviewed in some detail the performance and problems of the various persons for whom we were responsible. The same group[1] had voluntarily submitted to a battery of psychological tests conducted over a period of one academic year. You could argue the results two ways, I suppose. On one hand, the tests

---

[1] Permanent Deacon Class, Orchard Lake Center for Pastoral Studies, 1969-70.

came to pretty much the conclusions that we did and so you can say that the tests were accurate. On the other hand, you would have to say that we came to these conclusions without the help of the tests. Perhaps we were a little bit better off because we had not one standard but two. However, given the choice, I think a great many of us would prefer the considered judgment of competent persons over a period of time to exhaustive testing.

All of this, however, leads us away from the most important thing under consideration in this chapter and that is the right to privacy of every person and the right to protection of natural and committed secrets and any confidential information that is exchanged in the conduct of professional activities. It seems that our whole society needs a great big lesson in this area. If a lesson is not learned soon, we may be in for genuine disaster. Terrible abuses are carried out in the name of security or the welfare of the person himself or the overall efficiency of the organization. Granting that the common good sometimes has to supersede individual rights, allowing of this should take place only when one is absolutely sure of necessity and of proportionate cause. We seem to live in a time when our principle recreation is exchanging rather delicate information about one another. The Church certainly has a very plain role in discouraging this kind of activity. The sooner we get about it the better.

12. The Shrink Thing, Addicts, Abusers, and Punitive Treatment

Perhaps as good a way as any to begin this chapter is to quote what I used to call the Jacobian Dictum: Professional help doesn't necessarily.

For a long time, and the situation will probably continue for a long time, there has been a rather strong tendency in most parts of society to refer anyone manifesting difficult behavior at any level to someone connected with the psychiatric, psychological or psychiatric social work fields. It has been a natural enough development. The sudden and comprehensive insights in the general psychiatric field which began with the work of Sigmund Freud have offered hope where formerly there appeared to be none. However, as in all good things, the matter has been overdone and it is an area in which the average priest is going to find considerable difficulty if he takes his work seriously.

First of all, it must be noted that one of the most important things for both the physician and the priest is to be able to recognize behavior which calls for psychiatric investigation if not necessarily long-term therapy. There is little point in trying to treat by medication a condition which is largely emotional in origin. Similarly, the best intended pastoral counseling can actually be harmful in a case where the specific techniques of the psychiatric trade are called for. It would be very hard to state ground rules for deciding when a psychiatric referral should be made. Perhaps the best approach is to look at it the other way around and to say that while one must be very careful of extensive dealing with a patient or client who needs psychiatric care, at the present time there is probably more harm done by referring people who don't really need it.

Obvious psychotic or near psychotic behavior leaves little room for doubt. The mere fact that someone is a little bit confused and a little bit temperamental is not automatically a reason for calling for psychiatric consultation. The difficulty is that a great number of people who are well short of any line that might be called psychotic can actually be harmed by picking up some of the routine insights that come with psychiatric interviewing and counseling. There is nothing magic about it. The work of the same therapist on two people with roughly equal conditions may have widely varying results. Psychiatry is not now and probably never will be a very precise science.

Therefore, its use as an evasion for trying to handle relatively normal human problems may in some cases amount to an absolute evil. There are people for whom too much insight is a very bad thing. They may go along in a relatively normal manner, being just vaguely disturbed one way or another, but basically functioning and able to make some improvement with good advice and encouragement from a physician or a priest. The same people may be set back badly by the wrong psychiatric handling or by any psychiatric handling for that matter.

I am not knocking the psychiatric profession, merely pleading that it be treated with proper respect. There has been a tendency to send just about anybody who is difficult to deal with to the nearest psychiatrist or psychologist. Within the "shrink" profession, perhaps there has been too much willingness to take on just about any case that comes along.

One of the great difficulties is a proliferation of agencies and what we might call parapsychiatric personnel. A psychiatrist is an M.D. with specialized postgraduate training and experience in dealing with the emotionally disturbed and mentally ill. No one else is a psychiatrist. No one else should be called one. A clinical psychologist, practicing somewhat on the same level as a psychiatrist, should be called a psychologist and should have a doctorate if he is going to engage in the business of diagnosis and therapy. Persons with lesser qualifications in psychology may be of great help in a clinical situation. However, there is a great tendency in certain quarters to confuse not only patients but persons making referrals. Not long ago I sent a young man to an agency who told me that a psychiatrist would be available to see him at 8:00 the next morning. He wound up talking to a fellow with a master's degree in psychology whose experience had been pretty much limited to working with disturbed children. Needless to say, no one was very happy about the results.

Our beginning recommendations, then, are to be sure to make a psychiatric referral if there is strong evidence that this is called for, to avoid making psychiatric referrals merely to get rid of difficult persons, and to be very sure just whom we are dealing with in making referrals and recommending treatment. A psychiatrist may refer a case on to a clinical psychologist or, in a great many places, a clinical psychologist with proper certification may do the next thing to practicing medicine within the behavioral areas. Below this we have an unstratified area of counselors and social workers whose qualifications vary greatly. As noted, they may make monumental contributions from time to time, but should be called what they are. It seems to me that there is some genuinely unethical activity going on in giving the impression that various persons within a health care facility are more qualified than they are.

A quick answer to this is that you don't have to be a psychiatrist to help your brother. I would be the first to agree. In fact, some of the finest psychiatrists are recommending routine therapy handled by people with relatively little in the way of formal training. However, such therapy is overseen and directed by highly qualified persons. So called "group psychiatry" or "social psychiatry" has done a great deal for people with marginal troubles and should certainly be encouraged. However, it is just as unethical to refer a patient who thinks he is seeing a psychiatrist to a minimally qualified psychologist as it would be to send a difficult obstetrical case to a practical nurse with an unusual interest in midwifery.

Within the field of psychiatric treatment there are many grave ethical questions, some of which have caused the Church to look somewhat unfavorably on a lot of psychiatric activity. On the whole, the difficulties may have been exaggerated, but they do exist. The priest needs to give a great deal of thought to all sides of the question before taking a position. For instance, many in the Church are disturbed by the heavy interest shown by many in the psychiatric field in sexual fantasy and sexual activity. The interest is really quite legitimate, the problem is what do they do with it?

That is to say, there is nothing automatically unethical or immoral about investigating the sexual phase of one's life. After all, it is one of the major phases of life for any one of us. The difficulties that present themselves are excessive interest in this side of things and, more commonly, advice in certain directions which may seem to be in direct conflict with good moral counseling.

Here, you pretty much have to take it on a case-by-case basis. For instance, the therapist just as the confessor or spiritual director may "take it easy" for a long time in dealing with someone with a problem of habitual masturbation. Various things in the person's background and make-up may make it quite plain that a simple demand to stop such activity would be not only impossible to fulfill, but might cause worse trouble. This, as noted, is in the best tradition of pastoral counseling and would cause no real problems for a moralist.

There would be quite a difference, however, if the therapist gave the impression that he was approving masturbation, flatly stating that it was nothing to worry about or in some way giving the patient the impression that there was no moral question involved. It's very possible that the patient may not even be able to recognize what is meant by moral question and the therapist is not strictly obligated to get into it. What we are talking about is the difference between tolerating a certain practice and approving or appearing to approve of it if the practice is normally considered to be immoral.

A psychiatrist, like a good pastoral counselor, may be quite sympathetic with one who is trying to end an adulterous relationship and is having difficulty in doing so. Again, this is quite understandable and a lot of individual judgment has to be exercised. Merely piling up feelings of guilt or demanding behavior which is almost humanly impossible in a given situation will do little good to anyone. On the other hand, should the therapist give the impression that he views adulterous behavior as perfectly all right, we have an ethical problem. Worse yet is the case where the therapist, and this happens more often than you might think, flatly advises a patient to seek more and more varied sexual outlets.

A homosexual may have extreme difficulty, even with the best of good intentions, in totally avoiding homosexual activity. People in the pastoral and moral fields may argue the degrees and questions and circles involved at great length, but the fact remains that a true homosexual is not going to stop being one over night. This again, is a little different from simply giving a blanket approval to homosexuality or to any other practice or way of life generally considered to be immoral.

Within the Church there has been quite a tendency to be more tolerant of homosexuals and to urge those whose condition is seen to be virtually unchangeable to direct their activities toward deep and lasting relationships. I am not going to try to argue that one at this point, but merely make it clear that there are many ways of approaching the situation. As far as out and out medical ethics, about all the priest needs to have firmly in mind is that it is one thing to be open, accepting and nonjudgmental in dealing with the behavioral problem. It is quite another thing to recommend behavior which within Church circles would normally be classed as a moral problem.

I'm not going to try to put down any list of dos or don'ts or rights or wrongs because the entire area is terribly confused. There is, however, a certain faction within the psychiatric field which believes that just about anything can be cured with a little more sex. It's a charming notion to some, but one which should be looked at as carefully as one looks at freewheeling surgery. There are even cases where therapists have offered their own services in relieving the sexual anxieties of some of their patients, contrary to traditional professional ethics, regardless of the religious aspects of the situation. Nevertheless, the matter is not a completely uncommon one.

Sexual therapy in which individuals but more often partners are aided in overcoming difficulties and increasing the quality of their sexual performance is becoming more common. In certain cases it could be highly beneficial, but it now ranges from the highly controlled and extremely professional to pure quackery with all degrees in between. Further, the particular philosophies of the therapists vary considerably.

Right now the frequency of such treatment is limited, principally by the cost, which can be eighty dollars per hour or more over extended periods. However, it is virtually certain to become more common.

Where it is aimed at improving sex within marriage, it could be both moral in intent and have far-reaching moral consequences of a high nature. Such treatment is usually given to the couple as a couple and so long as they are aware of their sexual rights as a married couple there seems to be little reason to counsel against sexual therapy.

In cases where such counseling would not inhibit the parties unduly, the best course appears to be for the priest to discuss it with them from time to time as much for purposes of encouragement as to keep a reasonable eye open for indications of instructions or practices that could lead to moral damage and in many cases work against the treatment where it involves persons of good conscience and intention. For instance, some practitioners are said to employ "in-bed therapists," anonymous sexual partners who offer instruction and development "on location" as it were.

Whether we're talking about the use of drugs, compulsive stealing or just about any other activity which raises a moral question, the therapist may have to be quite tolerant of things which would normally be viewed as intolerable. So long as he does this with the intention of bringing about the correction of anti-social or immoral behavior with the overall best interests of the patient in mind, it would be hard to criticize him except on the basis of individual judgment in an individual instance. The same kind of very careful procedure with a given problem may have to be exercised by a priest any hour of the day or night. The only principle that seems to be consistent is that there is a distinction between accepting a person engaged in immoral activity and encouraging a person to seek or continue immoral activity indefinitely.

This could lead us through the whole range of sensitivity training and various subpsychiatric activities which have been quite common in our time. These vary so much that it seems impossible to lay down any flat code except that it seems quite likely that any priest of good background and good sense is going to know the difference between making a man a little freer and a little happier with daily living and daily contact with other persons and turning him on to the point where he kicks over the traces as far as reasonably acceptable social and moral conduct are involved.

Another ethical problem arises in the matter of confinement for purposes of psychiatric care. There is no doubt that within our time a great deal of this kind of confinement has been a little less than a racket. In the better psychiatric circles today, the tendency seems to be to get the patient moving as quickly as possible and to have him face his problems in a situation as close as possible to the one in which he will normally live. In other words, the old-time custodial care is very much out as far as psychiatrists are concerned. Still, there is a lot of it on both the government hospital level and on the private level and it would have to come down to a case of examining things instance by instance in order to make any kind of pronouncement as to the ethics of a situation.

One thing is certain: there is very little ethical justification for experimenting on a human being just because he is badly disturbed mentally. The same principles laid down in the chapter on human experimentation in general apply here, or perhaps we should say should apply here, but there seems to be a little bit more freewheeling experimentation on psychiatric cases than on others.

Free and easy treatment with any drug or any kind of therapy that comes along is the order of the day in many places, and this is pretty much unethical on the face of it. An area which bothers a lot of people is that of shock therapy. Although there is considerable theoretical material available, I have yet to see anything which states very plainly what shock therapy does, why and how. This being the case, it would have to be observed at the very least that such therapy is probably used a lot more than it should be.

In the matter of psychosurgery, we have another very delicate set of problems. There are surgeons who have been able to alter psychiatric conditions considerably, but in general, results of brain surgery aimed at correcting psychiatric conditions have been unpredictable and in some cases very, very dangerous. I am still haunted by the face of a doctor who was himself a patient in a state hospital in the 1940's. He had been a schizophrenic with paranoid tendencies who had been subjected to a lobotomy—cutting into the pre-frontal lobes of the brain with the aim of altering behavior. The result was that he was classified for the rest of his life as a schizophrenic of the hebephrenic[1] variety. To put it mildly, psychosurgery has a long way to go before it can be considered an ordinary means of approaching a situation. Even so, it cannot be ruled out completely, and if a priest is consulted in a given case about the only thing he can do is investigate the matter from all sides and come up with the best possible judgment. Extreme caution is in order.

Of course the big word in the whole field of antisocial behavior is drug abuse, including alcohol abuse.

Psychiatry as a field has not had a great deal to offer, although there is every reason to believe that there may be some breakthroughs before too long. The per-

---

[1] A kind of catch-all classification for patients who are vague, sometimes childish, perhaps a little unpredictable, somewhat vegetable-like.

son who is addicted to any drug or alcohol is certainly to be seen as a very sick person, although not necessarily a psychiatric patient. A psychiatric evaluation would seem to be pretty much routine for anyone in this category, but experience has shown that for most addicts, psychiatry alone does not hold the answer. A sympathetic physician, backed up by a social worker, clergyman, or any of a number of other possible sources may be able to accomplish quite a bit, but there are very few general rules in the field. Whether, for instance, drug addiction should be treated by switching the addict from one drug to another, is quite a question. It doesn't appear that it is an out and out moral question at this point. If a person could be cured of heroin addiction by judicious use of methadone, or any other drug for that matter, the procedure appears to be ethical and desirable. There are no completely convincing figures in the matter, but there are plenty of supporters of this kind of therapy.

Various kinds of withdrawal and rehabilitation programs have been increasing, happily, and a fair amount of success has been reported. Unfortunately, on the whole, the drug or alcohol abuser falls in the class of the very difficult patient whose prognosis is almost always somewhat questionable.

This is only a personal opinion, although it would be shared by thousands of persons, but the most effective thing available to most alcoholics seems to be Alcoholics Anonymous. Many psychiatrists have questioned its philosophy and approach, and they are certainly entitled to do this, but the fact remains that it has sobered up an awful lot of drunks and has kept some of the worst alcoholics sober for 15, 20, 25 years and even more. The Alcoholics Anonymous rate of improvement certainly is superior to the rate of improvement reported by any other source that I know of.

It is not infallible and never will be. Not every person will find his answer in AA. But speaking from a strictly pastoral point of view, it seems that anyone with a drinking problem should be urged to look into Alcoholics Anonymous and if possible at least give it a try. The organization does not force anyone to continue membership and makes no demands on him. It simply presents him with certain information and invites him to come along. It's pretty hard to beat that approach to anything. It seems to be necessary for the person to be at rock bottom one way or another in order for him to make the kind of decision which is the beginning of a successful membership in AA, but that rock bottom varies a great deal from person to person. One man may have to go all the way to Skid Row for ten years. Another may hit his own kind of "bottom" while still retaining an executive position and a good reputation in the community.

Various alcoholism treatment centers offer all kinds of approaches to the problem and, again, the racket has to be watched for. However, there are some institutions which do a good job of putting an alcoholic in reasonable physical and mental condition, helping him make the transition from an intoxicated life to a sober life and providing him with sufficient support as he gradually reenters the mainstream of society. Generally, these have been the least expensive programs, at least for the patient himself.

There are a couple of other moral points that need to be stressed very heavily. The Church and a great many of its institutions will simply have to take the blame for being backward in many places in approaching drug and alcohol abuse. I still know of Catholic hospitals that will not admit an alcoholic patient. If a man is important enough in the community he may be admitted under some other diagnosis, but an out-and-out alcoholic is simply not welcome. The same thing is true of the drug addict. It must be said that some of these hospitals don't have ideal facilities for treating alcoholics or addicts, but they get behavioral problems of other kinds and without very much trouble could equip themselves efficiently to deal with such cases as they arise. To put it in the strongest, plainest terms: An alcoholic or an addict is an honestly sick person. He can be helped and he is worth helping. That is an old cliche, but one which is not apt to be refuted in a hurry.

A great many physicians have an intense dislike for alcoholic and addictive patients and perhaps it's just as well that they don't deal with them. However, anything smacking of abuse or a failure to recognize human dignity in the person of an alcoholic or an addict is certainly in the area of questionable ethical conduct. This is true whether it is on the part of an individual practitioner or of an institution.

Within our hospitals another problem often arises. The alcoholic or addict may find himself treated in a punitive manner by some or many of the hospital personnel. In general, he is not taken as seriously as a straight medical patient and is talked about in a way which would violate a great many of the things that we mentioned in the previous chapter. A great many nurses and other personnel who deal from time to time with alcoholics and addicts have had unfortunate experiences in their own lives with drinkers and perhaps with drug users. I know of altogether too many cases where this kind of background has led to out-and-out punishment of patients, refusal to give them drugs as ordered, or just generally mean and unreasonable treatment of human persons. This is certainly outside of ethical bounds and the administration of any health care facility certainly has an obligation to watch for this kind of behavior and to take corrective measures wherever it appears. It may be as simple as transferring a nurse to another floor, but it should not be ignored. If a physician has ordered a certain drug for a patient, knowing that the patient is an addict or an alcoholic, the drug should be administered as ordered. If a nurse has any questions on the matter, the most that she can do ethically is call the situation to the doctor's attention and make sure that he intends the order, having a full understanding of the patient's background. Cases I know of where the nurse simply refused to give the medication would be very hard to justify. She is, in effect, practicing medicine without a license in addition to a number of other offenses which may be involved.

The great difficulty with alcoholism and drug addiction is that they rarely yield quickly to therapeutic measures and may continue for many months or many years without any outward sign of improvement. This is no reason to make any adverse moral judgment toward the patient. His morality is a thing apart, to be judged, in the final analysis, only by God, to be examined and perhaps discussed with a qualified clergyman or some other counselor. In no case is he less important, less human or less deserving of compassionate treatment than any other patient.

One of the good sides of the alcohol-drug situation is that occasionally there are rather dramatic improvements. Just what brings them about is hard to say, but people who have had severe alcohol or drug problems for a long time have been known to "snap out of it" rather suddenly, seek appropriate treatment and go on to live useful, normal lives. That certainly is worth hanging on for.

The priest in his day-to-day activities will probably have more trouble with the families of such patients than he will with the patients themselves. About all he can do is offer sympathy and support along with as much insight as possible to the condition involved. The sufferer will rarely seek his help except as a balm for a disturbed conscience or perhaps as a means of obtaining a little money. He will, however, benefit from anything positive and understanding that the priest does for him.

The ethics of the situations we have considered in this chapter are not clear-cut, but that is the whole purpose of the chapter. They range all the way from exercising care not to overrate psychiatry to being sure not to neglect psychiatry when it is called for. It is not always easy to know what is called for. There is every reason to believe that alcohol and drug problems will get a lot worse before they get better and the priest is probably going to play a major role in the situation as time goes on. The more he can keep himself informed, the better off everyone will be. The main thing seems to come down to the oft-recommended policy of being open, accepting and nonjudgmental. What really is called for in dealing with most emotional problems and especially with addictive problems is endless patience. Few of us were born with that, but most of us can at least try to cultivate it. More than once, an alcoholic or an addict or a severe neurotic with an apparently hopeless situation was helped primarily by the fact that a couple of people simply would not give up.

If there is any area in the health care field in which Christian mercy and compassion are called for and in which all of the normal virtues seem to be needed while being strained to the utmost, this is it.

Over the years, various members of the Church have made some mighty contributions to the field in general and to individual cases. A great deal more seems to be needed and anyone with the time and patience and good will to have a go at it will certainly find plenty of opportunity to put his services to the test.

Moral evaluations of the attitudes and activities of those in the psychiatric profession and related fields will have to be watched very carefully and very continuously. They do have a tendency to change.

At the present time many of the people working as psychologists, psychiatric social workers, and so forth, have a general philosophy of life which is considerably at odds with a traditional Catholic perspective and even more importantly with even a vaguely Christian perspective. Sizing up that situation is going to be a real headache for any priest and I only wish that I could offer more guidelines, but I have found them nowhere and I don't expect to.

13. Minds Get Made Up

For all the hurry, scurry and worry involved, minds do get made up on pastoral situations involving medical care. As long as the Church functions in anything like its present form—and we can presume that will be for quite a while—the man in the pastoral role will be asked to sit in on the discussions, to offer opinions, perhaps even to make a final judgment. I don't think there is anyone who has seriously considered the whole situation who would want him to do just that—make a final judgment.

Traditionally in morality we have taught that an action becomes fully moral only when one has studied the alternatives, studied the formal teachings on the matter, earnestly sought good advice, made a decision and then really made that decision his own so that the action flowing from the decision carries with it the fullness of morality.

In practice we haven't always operated that way and there are many reasons for it. For instance, for a long time priests felt that the main job was to pass on the formal teaching of the Church and to make that as palatable as possible. Sometimes they did this in cases where they knew the teaching would be followed to the letter, sometimes they did it when they knew that it would be ignored completely. In neither case could we say that a good pastoral solution had been found. The one followed out of a kind of blind obedience lacked something of real morality, real Christianity. The decision made in simple opposition to the formal teaching of the Church almost always carried with it at least an objective kind of immorality and, perhaps, a set of attitudes which kept the persons involved from ever seeking good pastoral counseling again.

What I am going to say here, then, may offend some and it may lead a few others to bend too far. After all, I can't form your conscience or do your job any more than you can form my conscience or do my job. I can only take the approach that seems best to me in the present time, given present conditions, and given the fullness and, if you will, the eternity of the faith.

Someone will remark if he has not already done so that for all of our talk about new directions in morality a great number of the cases come down to sex or reproduction in one form or another and we have already said that our ethics and morality must rise above the umbilicus. Still, on the pastoral level, the couple coming for counseling, even the individual, more often than not will have a problem which is related in some manner to sex or reproduction and in spite of all of our talk of the brave new world of medicine and experimental biology, a great deal of that, too, is closely tied to matters of sex and reproduction.

So what is one to do? The only solid suggestion I could make is the suggestion that is constantly made to teachers of theology and that is to be very sure that in dealing with the given situation one distinguishes plainly between formal, traditional teaching of the Church where that exists, theological opinion if that exists, and personal opinion where one chooses to express it. If he does this along with the sincere Christian love that should go into any counseling process, he can't go too far wrong. I do believe he would be wrong if he failed to cite something in canon law that didn't quite go along with the decision he felt should be made. I feel that he would be wrong in totally ignoring the Bishops' guidelines even though there is a great deal that could be said against them. Where it is a theological or legal matter that has to be explained in terms of its weight, he must be particularly careful even at the risk of being pedantic. If he does it, however, does it warmly, openly and, in cases where it is painful, lets it be known that it is painful to him, he will have taught something very important.

He will have taught that we do have a tradition, that we do have a heritage, that we do not take it lightly, that we never simply spit in its face. There are times when consciences can be directed in a pastoral situation which would lead quite a distance from what the flat, well-preserved teaching of the Church would urge. It may happen. Almost certainly it has happened to any man who has done any counseling at all. Really all he can do is work very hard on his own conscience and on his own prayer life and make sure that insofar as possible he is trying to speak as a representative of Christ, not only Christ the judge, but Christ the healer, Christ the lover of men. If an individual or a couple seeking aid sees this love reflected in the pastoral counselor, it simply has to have a weight, an influence, and a bearing, however imperceptible, in the final moral quality of the decision.

The trouble is, and I think most priests know this, that they are approached very frequently by people who ask questions in apparent innocence but whose minds have really been made up, who are already in a situation or committed to get into a situation which will put them flatly at odds with the Church. If the counselor is convinced that this is the case all he can do is try to fit their decision into a Christian framework, argue with his best talents for a Christian framework, but to make sure that in any case if they have to go away without any formal sign of approval from the formal Church that they go away also knowing that Christ loves them and that if somehow they err or sin Christ can and will forgive them if they so desire.

The great problem is that the Church doesn't know a great deal about medicine. Medicine doesn't know a great deal about medicine right now and as we've said repeatedly in these pages, new situations, developments, procedures will continue to arise and these in themselves are of an abstract sort that don't fully enter into the human until they begin to be the treatment of a person or persons. There are no two identical persons and there are no two identical situations. So without wanting to sound like a moral anarchist of some sort we must say that there probably are no two identical answers.

One of the things that we have to face most strongly is the notion rooted so deeply in so many that the Church has the final word on everything. The other thing we have to face is a notion rooted very firmly in at least as many and perhaps more that the Church really has nothing to say about anything, that one could feel a little bit more at ease in conscience if he had the blessing of the Church in a situation, but, in the final analysis, that it was the human need that had to be met, the human tension that had to be stopped, the human situation that had to be solved.

This places upon the back of the counselor a real share of the cross of Christ himself. He simply cannot know enough to be an answer man, he can only do this. He can make sure first of all that he knows the people, that he knows them as well as possible and as any experienced priest counselor will tell you that doesn't usually happen on the first session or the second or the third. He has to be careful that he's not projecting his own needs and feelings into theirs or identifying their situation with one which has affected his life in some way. He has to be terribly sure that he has the best medical information possible. This is easier and easier to come by. Most teaching hospitals and medical schools will go out of their way to aid a clergyman who sincerely desires to know what the options and the probabilities are in a given situation. His knowledge, of course, may go way beyond that. It may go into the deepest part of the lives of those whom he counsels. It must, in spite of itself, be concerned more than with the immediate and yet it must not let some future misty untheologically settled goal be a reason for a command or a prohibition which may result in real human harm.

He must be careful not to worship medicine and its personnel. He must be careful not to be overwhelmed by its progress. He must be careful not to be shocked by its mistakes and its inadequacies and its corruption.

As in any other phase of pastoral life, he must be a man of tremendous breadth, of tremendous sensitivity. He must be the kind of man from whom a couple will walk away having been counseled against that which they have decided to do and still be very sure that he loves them, that he cares for them, that they are welcome back. He must be very sure no one ever despairs of the love and the forgiveness of Christ.

It is axiomatic that the pastoral disciplines will not keep up with the clinical disciplines in the days to come nor will they even be able to always be sure that they really know what goes on in any given household. I was shocked recently to learn that some editors thought I was out of touch with family life and I had been living a family life all the time. But perhaps they were right. Perhaps the nature of my own life, the place in which I live it, the way in which I live it, have put me out of touch with the great majority of people who live, move and have their being in a world so perplexing and so unceasing in its questions, its problems and its pressures that no one man has a chance of survival without a close consciousness of the presence of Christ.

I dealt recently with a case which involves father, mother, daughter, teenage son and two younger children. There is an extremely difficult set of decisions to be made, there is unbelievable suffering. I cannot solve, alone or even with a lot of the help that's available to me, all of the problems of just this one family. All I can know for sure is that the problems will continue, that they probably will get worse. What I have to communicate is that somehow, at its most unbearable, life has meaning because God is and because God is in Christ and because God in Christ is approachable by any man who will approach him even when there are no plain answers, even when the obvious clinical and pastoral alternatives seem to be exhausted.

So perhaps when the man or the woman who after pastoral counseling walks away into what looks like a blacker despair than ever and the heart of the priest sinks deeper than ever, almost drowning in its own inadequacy, almost despairing of the power of prayer to aid it, perhaps it is then that we come closest to touching Christ. It wouldn't be easy to tell patients that. It never will be.

I have found, though, that they do respond to honest recognition of that even when it leaves the counselor and the counselee with decisions that they simply cannot share except in the sense of humans caring for one another.

Fortunately, it's not always that black. There are the wonderful chances to carry the finest kind of morality, the finest kind of Christianity into any hospital ward or any sick room any time at all where one's simple presence may mean more than anyone could ever explain and where there is a real chance to laugh or share some new joy. It would be very easy for anyone doing much pastoral work in a medical setting to become bitter or cynical or flippant or, worse yet, really hardened. This is the only thing approaching real sin I can think of. So long as he can keep his original fresh hope in the redemption and in the resurrection and as long as he can communicate his own closeness to that, he is never failing whatever the final decisions are.

We will almost certainly never see a time again when the Church will simply say, "yes you can do this, no you can't do that" and have people act accordingly. People aren't growing up that way anymore. There is little reason to think that they will. For some reason, though, an awful lot of them still care and the one thing they will always respond to is caring. Caring is the one thing the priest can always give.

Again, as I have said so many times, it would be so nice to wind up with flat directives about how to sort out and evaluate the alternatives and to guide always toward the right one. You know and I know that day is gone, that in a real sense, if you want to be reflective enough, it never existed. We just thought it did. What the priest can take to the patient is Christ in himself, what he can take from the patient is Christ in the patient. Put it together, you wind up with Christ, despite confusion, despair, ultimate complexity. That's enough. God walk with you.

Appendix

ETHICAL AND RELIGIOUS DIRECTIVES
FOR CATHOLIC HEALTH FACILITIES

PREAMBLE

Catholic health facilities witness to the saving presence of Christ and His Church in a variety of ways: by testifying to transcendent spiritual beliefs concerning life, suffering and death; by humble service to humanity and especially to the poor; by medical competence and leadership; and by fidelity to the Church's teachings while ministering to the good of the whole person.

The total good of the patient, which includes his higher spiritual as well as his bodily welfare, is the primary concern of those entrusted with the management of a Catholic health facility. So important is this, in fact, that if an institution could not fulfill its basic mission in this regard, it would have no justification for continuing its existence as a Catholic health facility. Trustees and administrators of Catholic health facilities should understand that this responsibility affects their relationship with every patient, regardless of religion, and is seriously binding in conscience.

A Catholic-sponsored health facility, its board of trustees, and administration face today a serious difficulty as, with community support, the Catholic health facility exists side by side with other medical facilities not committed to the same moral code, or stands alone as the one facility serving the community. However, the health facility identified as Catholic exists today and serves the community in a large part because of the past dedication and sacrifice of countless individuals whose lives have been inspired by the Gospel and the teachings of the Catholic Church.

And just as it bears responsibility to the past, so does the Catholic health facility carry special responsibility for the present and future. Any facility identified as Catholic assumes with this identification the responsibility to reflect in its policies and practices the moral teachings of the Church, under the guidance of the local Bishop. Within the community the Catholic health facility is needed as a courageous witness to the highest ethical and moral principles in its pursuit of excellence.

The Catholic-sponsored health facility and its board of trustees, acting through its chief executive officer, further carry an overriding responsibility in conscience to prohibit those procedures which are morally and spiritually harmful. The basic norms delineating this moral responsibility are listed in these Ethical and Religious Directives for Catholic Health Facilities. It should be understood that patients and those who accept board membership, staff appointment or privileges, or employment in a Catholic health facility will respect and agree to abide by its policies and these Directives. Any attempt to use a Catholic health facility for procedures contrary to these norms would indeed compromise the board and administration in its responsibility to seek and protect the total good of its patients under the guidance of the Church.

These Directives prohibit those procedures which, according to present knowledge, are recognized as clearly wrong. The basic moral absolutes which underlie these Directives are not subject to change, although particular applications might be modified as scientific investigation and theological development open up new problems or cast new light on old ones.

In addition to consultations among theologians, physicians, and other medical and scientific personnel in local areas, the Committee on Health Affairs of the United States Catholic Conference, with the widest consultation possible, should regularly receive suggestions and recommendations from the field, and should periodically discuss any possible need for an updated revision of these Directives.

The moral evaluation of new scientific developments and legitimately debated questions must be finally submitted to the teaching authority of the Church in the person of the local Bishop, who has the ultimate responsibility for teaching Catholic doctrine.

SECTION I:
ETHICAL AND RELIGIOUS DIRECTIVES

1. The procedures listed in these Directives as permissible require the consent at least implied or reasonably presumed, of the patient or his guardians. This condition is to be understood in all cases.

2. No person may be obliged to take part in a medical or surgical procedure which he judges in conscience to be immoral; nor may a health facility or any of its staff be obliged to provide

a medical or surgical procedure which violates their conscience or these Directives.

3. Every patient, regardless of the extent of his physical or psychic disability, has a right to be treated with a respect consonant with his dignity as a person.

4. Man has the right and the duty to protect the integrity of his body together with all of its bodily functions.

5. Any procedure potentially harmful to the patient is morally justified only insofar as it is designed to produce a proportionate good.

6. Ordinarily the proportionate good that justifies a medical or surgical procedure should be a total good of the patient himself.

7. Adequate consultation is recommended, not only when there is doubt concerning the morality of some procedure, but also with regard to all procedures involving serious consequences, even though such procedures are listed here as permissible.

8. Everyone has the right and the duty to prepare for the solemn moment of death. Unless it is clear, therefore, that a dying patient is already well-prepared for death as regards both spiritual and temporal affairs, it is the physician's duty to inform him of his critical condition or to have some other responsible person impart this information.

9. The obligation of professional secrecy must be carefully fulfilled not only as regards the information on the patient's charts and records but also as regards confidential matters learned in the exercise of professional duties. Moreover,

the charts and records must be duly safeguarded against inspection by those who have no right to see them.

10. The directly intended termination of any patient's life, even at his own request, is always morally wrong.

11. From the moment of conception, life must be guarded with the greatest care. Any deliberate medical procedure, the purpose of which is to deprive a fetus or an embryo of its life, is immoral.

12. Abortion, that is, the directly intended termination of pregnancy before viability, is never permitted nor is the directly intended destruction of a viable fetus. Every procedure whose sole immediate effect is the termination of pregnancy before viability is an abortion, which, in its moral context, includes the interval between conception and implantation of the embryo.

13. Operation, treatments, and medications, which do not directly intend termination of pregnancy but which have as their purpose the cure of a proportionately serious pathological condition of the mother, are permitted when they cannot be safely postponed until the fetus is viable, even though they may or will result in the death of the fetus. If the fetus is not certainly dead, it should be baptized.

14. Regarding the treatment of hemorrhage during pregnancy and before the fetus is viable: Procedures that are designed to empty the uterus of a living fetus still effectively attached to the mother are not permitted; procedures designed to stop hemorrhage (as distinguished from those

designed precisely to expel the living and attached fetus) are permitted insofar as necessary, even if fetal death is inevitably a side effect.

15. Cesarean section for the removal of a viable fetus is permitted, even with risk to the life of the mother, when necessary for successful delivery. It is likewise permitted, even with risk to the child, when necessary for the safety of the mother.

16. In extrauterine pregnancy the dangerously affected part of the mother (e.g. cervix, ovary, or fallopian tube) may be removed, even though fetal death is foreseen, provided that:

    (a) the affected part is presumed already to be so damaged and dangerously affected as to warrant its removal, and that

    (b) the operation is not just a separation of the embryo or fetus from its site within the part (which would be a direct abortion from a uterine appendage), and that

    (c) the operation cannot be postponed without notably increasing the danger to the mother.

17. Hysterectomy, in the presence of pregnancy and even before viability, is permitted when directed to the removal of a dangerous pathological condition of the uterus of such serious nature that the operation cannot be safely postponed until the fetus is viable.

SECTION II:
PROCEDURES INVOLVING REPRODUCTIVE
ORGANS AND FUNCTIONS

18. Sterilization, whether permanent or temporary,

for men or for women, may not be used as a means of contraception.

19. Similarly excluded is every action which, either in anticipation of the conjugal act, or in its accomplishment, or in the development of its natural consequences, proposes, whether as an end or as a means, to render procreation impossible.

20. Procedures that induce sterility, whether permanent or temporary, are permitted when: (a) they are immediately directed to the cure, diminution, or prevention of a serious pathological condition and are not directly contraceptive (that is, contraception is not the purpose); and (b) a simpler treatment is not reasonably available. Hence, for example, oophorectomy or irradiation of the ovaries may be allowed in treating carcinoma of the breast and metastasis therefrom; and orchidectomy is permitted in the treatment of carcinoma of the prostate.

21. Because the ultimate personal expression of conjugal love in the marital act is viewed as the only fitting context for the human sharing of the divine act of creation, donor insemination and insemination that is totally artificial are morally objectionable. However, help may be given to a normally performed conjugal act to attain its purpose. The use of the sex faculty outside the legitimate use by married partners is never permitted even for medical or other laudable purpose, e.g. masturbation as a means of obtaining seminal specimens.

22. Hysterectomy is permitted when it is sincerely judged to be a necessary means of removing

some serious uterine pathological condition. In these cases, the pathological condition of each patient must be considered individually and care must be taken that a hysterectomy is not performed merely as a contraceptive measure, or as a routine procedure after any definite number of Cesarean sections.

23. For a proportionate reason, labor may be induced after the fetus is viable.

24. In all cases in which the presence of pregnancy would render some procedure illicit (e.g. curettage), the physician must make use of such pregnancy tests and consultation as may be needed in order to be reasonably certain that the patient is not pregnant. It is to be noted that curettage of the endometrium after rape to prevent implantation of a possible embryo is morally equivalent to abortion.

25. Radiation therapy of the mother's reproductive organs is permitted during pregnancy only when necessary to suppress a dangerous pathological condition.

SECTION III:
OTHER PROCEDURES

26. Therapeutic procedures which are likely to be dangerous are morally justifiable for proportionate reasons.

27. Experimentation on patients without due consent is morally objectionable, and even the moral right of the patient to consent is limited by his duties of stewardship.

28. Euthanasia ("mercy killing") in all forms is forbidden. The failure to supply the ordinary means of preserving life is equivalent to euthanasia. However, neither the physician nor the patient is obliged to use extraordinary means.

29. It is not euthanasia to give a dying person sedatives and analgesics for the alleviation of pain, when such a measure is judged necessary, even though they may deprive the patient of the use of reason, or shorten his life.

30. The transplantation of organs from living donors is morally permissible when the anticipated benefit to the recipient is proportionate to the harm done to the donor, provided that the loss of such organ(s) does not deprive the donor of life itself nor the functional integrity of his body.

31. Post-mortem examinations must not be begun until death is morally certain. Vital organs, that is, organs necessary to sustain life, may not be removed until death has taken place. The determination of the time of death must be made in accordance with responsible and commonly accepted scientific criteria. In accordance with current medical practice, to prevent any conflict of interest, the dying patient's doctor or doctors should ordinarily be distinct from the transplant team.

32. Ghost surgery, which implies the calculated deception of the patient as to the identity of the operating surgeon, is morally objectionable.

33. Unnecessary procedures, whether diagnostic or therapeutic, are morally objectionable. A procedure is unnecessary when no proportionate reason justifies it. A fortiori, any procedure that

is contraindicated by sound medical standards
is unnecessary.

SECTION IV:
THE RELIGIOUS CARE OF PATIENTS

34. The administration should be certain that patients in a health facility receive appropriate spiritual care.

35. Except in cases of emergency (i.e., danger of death), all requests for baptism made by adults or for infants should be referred to the chaplain of the health facility.

36. If a priest is not available, anyone having the use of reason and proper intention can baptize. The ordinary method of conferring emergency baptism is as follows: the person baptizing pours water on the head in such a way that it will flow on the skin, and, while the water is being poured, must pronounce these words audibly: I baptize you in the name of the Father, and of the Son, and of the Holy Spirit. The same person who pours the water must pronounce the words.

37. When emergency baptism is conferred, the chaplain should be notified.

38. It is the mind of the Church that the sick should have the widest possible liberty to receive the sacraments frequently. The generous cooperation of the entire staff and personnel is requested for this purpose.

39. While providing the sick abundant opportunity to receive Holy Communion, there should be no

interference with the freedom of the faithful to communicate or not to communicate.

40. In wards and semi-private rooms, every effort should be made to provide sufficient privacy for confession.

41. When possible, one who is seriously ill should be given the opportunity to receive the Sacraments of the Sick, while in full possession of his rational faculties. The chaplain must, therefore, be notified as soon as an illness is diagnosed as being so serious that some probability of death is recognized.

42. Personnel of a Catholic health facility should make every effort to satisfy the spiritual needs and desires of non-Catholics. Therefore, in hospitals and similar institutions conducted by Catholics, the authorities in charge should, with the consent of the patient, promptly advise ministers of other communions of the presence of their communicants and afford them every facility for visiting the sick and giving them spiritual and sacramental ministrations.

43. If there is a reasonable cause present for not burying a fetus or member of the human body, these may be cremated in a manner consonant with the dignity of the deceased human body.

SOURCES

Final paragraph of Preamble: Vatican II, *Constitution on the Church, #27*

DIRECTIVE

3 *Pacem in Terris,* n. 11

11 Vatican II, *The Church in the Modern World*, n. 51

18 *Humanae Vitae*, n. 14

19 *Humanae Vitae*, n. 14

20 *Humanae Vitae*, n. 15

28 Vatican II, *The Church in the Modern World*, n. 27

42 Directory for the Application of the Decisions of the Second Ecumenical Council of the Vatican Concerning Ecumenical Matters, n. 63

43 *Canon Law Digest*, Vol. 6, p. 669